Low Carb Diet Mistakes You Wish You Knew

Mirsad Hasic

DEDICATION

I dedicate this book to my wife.

CONTENTS

ACKNOWLEDGMENTS

I would like to thank my family for their support.

1 LIFESTYLE CHANGE

Do you want to look and feel your very best? Are you tired of not having the energy you need to keep up with all of life's challenges? Do you just want to see something other than a lumpy physique in the mirror at every turn?

Don't worry if you're eagerly nodding your head. I wanted all of those things as well, and like most people, I thought a diet would bring me what I really wanted. It took me a little bit to realize that the diet will only get you so far.

Then, as diets are wont to do, it'll swing the other way, driving the pounds right back on. It's a vicious cycle, and I decided that it was time to break it. Instead of diet after diet, I realized that making a lifestyle change would be far more effective.

Thankfully, the science backs the idea of a lifestyle change over a diet. According to Dr. Pamela Peeke, MD, MPH, FACP, the very act of dieting is a stressor to the body, causing you to store more fat. Cortisol is the stress hormone responsible for this mechanism, as the body considers dieting a position where your body is slowly but surely being led to starvation. It's a survival reaction of the highest order, that's for sure. [1]

There's also evidence that both genders are definitely affected by stress when it comes to weight loss. I'm a man with my own share of life stress factors, but who isn't stressed these days? Still, a study from the American Journal of Epidemiology suggests that we need to curb stress in order to lose weight. [2]

Moving back to the idea of a lifestyle change, you have it in you. Going with a lower-carbohydrate approach is one of the best "middle of the road" approaches, since you aren't going to have to make huge sacrifices.

After all, low-carb doesn't mean low on flavor, low on energy, or low on taste. You can get a wide range of cuisines handled successfully on low-carb without feeling deprived. But what is low-carb dieting all about?

As the name suggests, it's about lowering carbohydrate intake. Generally speaking, you'll get at least a third of your calories from protein, which can be a significant shift away from the way you're eating currently.

For example, you might be eating mostly carbs at this point with very little protein. Not all protein is created equal as well -- the plant sources of protein don't quite measure up to all of the meat-based sources of protein. [3]

In order to get as low-carb as possible, you'll want to stick to whole foods. This means that giving up a lot of wheat and processed wheat products is a good thing. While you might miss that morning donut with your coffee, I can assure you that you will not want to miss the body transformation that's in store for you. As you start seeing results in the mirror, you'll actually wonder why you didn't start sooner.

Low-carb also focuses on getting a lot of veggies into your diet, along with plenty of protein. You want to reach for balance rather than going overboard on one thing. There's no reason why you can't enjoy a big, green salad alongside your steak, for instance. In the beginning, you'll want to stick to good sources of fat, protein, and veggies.

As you commit more to the lifestyle, you can pursue some low-carb desserts sparingly. It's all a matter of thinking about your goals. If you really want to focus on weight loss, you're going to have to think of a different reward besides ice-cream.

Just because something is low-carb doesn't mean that you need to necessarily eat it. It's merely there as an option instead of going back to higher-carbohydrate foods. You may find that as you change your lifestyle, you really have no need to go for desserts. Fat is very satisfying, even though it's not as nutrient dense as protein. [4]

It can be a long, aching road to a better life. That's why I created a guide filled with mistakes that tend to get made it when it comes to changing over to eating low-carb for life. It might not be easy, but it's definitely worth it. I believe that by focusing on what not to do, you can build a solid plan filled with things to stay "on track". This series covers the top forty mistakes, but you'll see definite connections between each one.

I am deeply committed to seeing each and every person who reads this embark on a journey that will change their health for the better. Could you imagine having less weight and more energy to chase the kids around?

2 NEW WAY OF EATING

If you liked the last tip, this one will be right up your alley. You see, one of the top mistakes people face when trying to go low carb is that they don't prepare for this new way of eating. In the last article, I mentioned how so many people end up destroying their health through destructive diet cycles.

This isn't about that -- it's about creating a new life through changing your eating habits for the long term. Anything less than that just doesn't make sense at all. You're much better off thinking about how you're going to actually put your low carb plan into action.

It all starts with your kitchen. If you're living with other people, this might get a little complicated. Basically, you need to be on Planet Low Carb as much as possible in the very beginning. I found that going completely low carb was the only way to go.

Trying to do half low carb and half high carb is a recipe for disaster. When you have an emotional moment, guess which type of food you're going to actually reach for? Hint: it won't be the low carb stuff. The high bursts of sugar may elevate your mood temporary, but that's all it is: a temporary high. Sugar also plays a known role in the development of Type 2 Diabetes. It's been shown that 8,000 out of every 100,000 people will become diabetic. [5]

Going back to the main subject, you really want to make sure that you're preparing your kitchen as much as possible. This way if you get hungry you're going to immediately head over to something that's on plan. Off plan foods have no place in your life anymore.

It was really hard for me to give up normal high sugar chocolate because I was used to rewarding myself with that. But have you ever considered that food wasn't meant to be that rewarding? [6]

Food is designed to keep you fueled and ready for the next hunt. We're a long way from hunting down large mammals, but our bodies still run on the same type of fuel.

Your kitchen will usually be divided into dry and cold storage areas. Everything in the cold storage section needs to be low carb, because that's where you're going to go most.

Your vegetables need to be stored in a crisper to stay fresh for as long as possible, and you'll also want to keep plenty of meat on hand. If you're someone that's incredibly busy like I am, why not cut up all of your meat and vegetables at the same time? It can all be stored in separate little containers.

When you're ready to cook with something, you can do that. When you're ready to throw something in the oven, everything is already measured out. This will save you a lot more time in the kitchen than you think it will.

Your dry area should help balance out your cold storage items. Spices, herbs, and flavorings can all enhance your dining experience. At first, you want to make sure that your low carb diet pleases you and nourishes you. This means getting plenty of fat in there.

Butter, ghee, tallow, lard, coconut oil and avocado oil can all be great sources of fat for you while you're on low carb. What you want to avoid is vegetable oil, canola oil, corn oil, peanut oil, and safflower oil. They turn rancid and spur the generation of free-radicals that damage the body from the inside out. [7]

Give yourself a chance to really look at the foods that you like to eat. If there are low carb versions of what you normally eat, you might want to go with those as a very short, very gentle introduction. It's completely up to you.

When I first began low carb, I realized what a crutch these "comfort foods" can be. If you can tear yourself off of the old stuff, do so. It might be painful in the short term, but it will be worth it in the long run.

Having a slow cooker will help you make multiple lunches and dinners so that it's one less thing you have to worry about. The slow cooker is very inexpensive and can be found just about anywhere.

Thinking about getting started? Don't just think about it -- sit down, make a list of great low-carb foods, and then go out there and fill up your kitchen. You can always let your family eat the things that are no longer part of your eating plan. Good luck!

3 CALORIE INTAKE

Excited about low carb? I'm glad you are -- when I first started, I was pumped about finally finding something that could lead me to better health. However, the road ahead of you won't be straightforward all the time.

You'll have challenges that you need to get through, and you're going to have to do it as people doubt your abilities. You're going to have to do it even when it's not the "right time" to think about yourself. Remember that you can't take care of anyone if your own health is compromised.

Moving to the topic, one of the next mistakes that I see people make quite often is ignoring their ideal caloric intake. So when they binge out of control with low carb foods, they often tell me that they don't understand why the pounds are creeping back in with a vengeance.

The reality? You're taking in too many calories, far more than what you need to maintain. Now you're growing outward again, and it feels dark, hopeless, and downright tiring. It doesn't have to be that way -- you just need to know your body a bit better. Let me explain.

A calorie is simply a unit of energy -- but it tells us how much energy it roughly takes to power to body's various processes. Even as you sleep, your body is repairing your tissues, forming new neural pathways, and otherwise being a well-run piece of machinery, so to speak. [8]

Figuring out how many calories you need can be tricky. There are quite a few different systems out there, and you might feel overwhelmed. I'm here to tell you that it's really not that complicated at all. Today's Internet users can easily find calorie requirement calculators just about everywhere. [9]

Most of them will ask you the basic bits of information, such as your height, age, gender, and weight. Not only that, it'll want to know how activate you really are. If you're someone that gets really active, then you're going to require more calories than someone that is fairly sedentary.

I was very much into soccer when I started low-carb, so I found myself selecting "moderate". You might go with sedentary if you really don't move around much. I can't tell you enough about the benefits of exercising, but it's up to you to actually go through with that. It's not like you have to work out in order to lose weight with a low carb lifestyle, but it does help.

The number that you get after you finish entering in your data may surprise you. For example, under the Harris Benedict Equation [2], a 35 year old man of average height [6' feet] and weight [200 pounds] who works out moderately would be looking at 2,918 as a basal metabolic rate.

This means that his body needs 2,918 to maintain regular functions. If you're trying to lose weight, you'll need to create an energy deficit. [3], [4].

This is where you will eat either fewer calories than what's needed, or raising the number of calories burned through exercise. You can also combine the two tactics together to make sure that you're losing a bit of weight consistently.

It's important to use a calculator to determine how many

calories your body actually burns in a given day. This is going to be an estimate, but it's better than nothing. From there, you can look at your activity level to figure out a ballpark figure for your calories.

Using the example I have earlier of the 35 year old man who burns 2918 calories a day, he may want to use exercise to give him a 500 calorie deficit, or eat fewer than 2918 calories. Over the course of a week, this does result in a slow but consistent weight loss pattern [10,11].

It can be confusing and frustrating at the beginning, and I know that you're going to feel like giving up. Don't give up right before you're able to get things done. Make sure that you break free and do what's right for you.

Once you have a good grasp of calories, you can begin planning your meals properly. What's that? You think that you don't need to plan your meals out as a new low carb follower? Guess we know which mistake is up next, eh?

4 NOT PLANNING MEALS

Well, I'm back with another mistake that you should avoid as you wade deeper and deeper into a low carb lifestyle. If I could highlight anything at this point, it would certainly be the need to make this a lifestyle.

All of these mistakes are designed to push you deeper into making this a habit that you keep and maintain for life, not just another diet that's going to eventually fail you.

Diets encourage you to get bored and leave them. Lifestyles encourage you to keep them forever. It's certainly up to you to figure out what you're going to choose but I know what I am going with. This is totally a lifestyle for me.

Anyway, let's move on to that mistake, shall we? Today's mistake is straightforward: you're just not planning your meals out. Do you know what you invite in when you don't plan your meals out?

You're inviting the chance of going off plan. In the first 90 days of going low carb, this is the last thing that you really want to do with your plan.

You can't just cheat at will. You have to be completely committed to it. There are really so many little things that can take your focus away from your new way of eating, and it's important to close off these holes of temptation when you can. [12]

What I like to do in order to prepare for low carb eating on the go is to take a cooler with me. Does it feel a little silly at first? Yes, it does but the alternative is worse -- I go and find the highest carb thing I can stuff into my mouth, therefore ruining my meal. It's far too easy to rationalize away bad eating.

You start thinking that the day is ruined and there's really no reason to mess around with anything on plan. So your brain, stimulated by the chance of getting foods that aren't suitable, goes into overdrive.

Without rules and structure, you feel free to eat anything that looks appealing to you. Never mind that you are going to be undoing progress that you've made. It's a short term fix to a long term problem that won't go away until you change your attitude. [13]

Preparing is more than just getting your kitchen ready -- it's getting your mind ready as well. You want to make sure that you're taking things with you everywhere you go. At home, you need to bring low carb snacks next to your desk.

If you have to hunt for something low carb, chances are good that you're going to skip the search and go for the easy. The key to making your lifestyle change stick is to realize that it's not about easy -- you have to just do things that you really don't want to do at first.

Going back to all of your reasons why you wanted to lose weight can help you avoid giving in to temptation. Other people have to go and look at visuals of themselves at a heavier weight than what they are at the current time.

Whatever method will help you stay on track the most effectively is the choice that you should make. Everyone's motivation is going to be different. As I told you before, my basic motivation was pretty vain. I wanted to look good -- to look even better than the day I got married.

I wanted to be fit and I wanted my wife to notice me

every time I walked into the room. You might want other people to notice your new size. You might want to prove to your parents that you don't have to spend the rest of your life being overweight and looked down upon by people that have never been overweight in their entire lives.

Holding yourself accountable can be absolutely difficult. Even though you know that low carb can lead you to the paradise you've always dreamed about, the reality is that a few words are enough to destroy the rest of your future.

I'm not trying to be over the top or anything like that, but it's really important that you start looking at the future you want, rather than the future that you'll have if your weight gets out of control.

I'm talking about all of the dangers of obesity -- heart disease, diabetes, gallstones, sleep apnea, strokes, high blood pressure, cholesterol ...the list goes on and on. [14]

Only you can make the right decisions over your own life, but I hope that my guides on what NOT to do with low carb eating means that you'll have it a bit easier in terms of figuring out which traditions to cherish, and which ones to skip over.

5 ENOUGH SLEEP

As you work your way through low carb eating, you might find that some of the struggles that you dealt with on the first day just aren't so awkward. You're no longer stopping dead in your tracks at the entrance of a grocery store, frozen with fear over whether or not they'll have food for you to eat.

The grocery store will have a lot of low carb goodies that are worth checking out. They just aren't always labeled low carb outright, so you might skip right over them. Cauliflower, squash, berries, and more are all foods that don't have a low carb label, but many low carb fans enjoy them.

You can also enjoy tomatoes, cucumbers, zucchini, spinach, kale, cabbage and even a few carrots. Low carb isn't so restrictive that you'll never see another leaf of Romaine lettuce or another onion.

You will be able to enjoy a wide variety of choices, but today's mistake isn't about food at all. It's something that low carbers tend to skip over quite a bit, even if their way of eating is nailed down properly.

The problem, in a nutshell: not enough sleep. Sleep is

absolutely essential if you're trying to lose weight on low carb. If you don't get sleep, you're going to have a stress reaction.

The body responds to lack of sleep by producing cortisol, which in turn signals the body to start storing fat again. (15) If you've taken all of the hard steps to change your lifestyle, you need to go a little farther by making your sleep a priority.

The first reply that I get out of a lot of people when I talk about sleep is how busy they are. Why do we wear our "business" as a badge of honor? Life wasn't supposed to be this challenging, and it's still not supposed to be so unfriendly.

Have you tried to get two people together to have a conversation that doesn't involve Facebook or LinkedIn or Twitter or even just text messaging? It's absolutely difficult, and it's just one little symptom of the bigger problem

I think our culture has: we want instant results. That's why the restaurants and health spas seem to be overflowing while the yoga practices seem to be dwindling.

If you're trying to slow down and really embrace low-carb, you have to think about sleeping more. Knowing how much to sleep can lead to a few different answers. According to the National Sleep Foundation, there's really no magic number that everyone corresponds to.

So if the average is 8 and you seem to thrive on 6, it's perfectly okay to enjoy those six hours. If you're someone that needs 10 hours instead of 8, there's no need to feel guilty that you really need more than other people. (16)

If you're looking for better sleep, I have plenty of tips for you on that subject. I struggled with insomnia for several years, but I never realized how much damage it did to me until I got older. It's harder to fall asleep when you've been awake for longer and longer hours, but it can be done.

You need to make sure that you're not just thinking about how long you stay asleep, but the type of sleep that you're getting. If you're never able to get comfortable then your sleep quality will not be very good at all. (17)

The best thing that you can do for your sleep is try to actually get consistent about it. Trying to have different bedtimes all throughout the week is going to just leave you feeling groggy and unmotivated when you finally have to get up. The last thing that you want to try to do is have every electronic device in existence plugged in and turned on where you can see them.

These little pinpricks of light might not sound like much, but they can actually disturb the body's natural sleep cycle, including that part of the night where you feel like you're gently being pulled to sleep. (18)

If you're going to still enjoy coffee and alcohol, you want to make sure that you enjoy them well before you're ready to actually go to bed. Even though alcohol is a depressant, it has been shown to affect sleep patterns tremendously. (19)

You are much better off making sure that you are going to have the right environment for sleep. Blocking out as much light as possible will also help with this, so you can get the rest you deserve.

Of course, we're nowhere near finished with the top mistakes I see people make when it comes to low carbing, but I figured you should know how to improve the quality of your sleep. Sleep is a very restorative process, and you need to get the highest quality of sleep you can get.

To do anything else would be to poison your body -- literally!

6 NOT ENOUGH PROTEIN

Well, I'm back to give you everything I can when it comes to following a low carb lifestyle filled with new food adventures, laughter, and fun. Life is too short to take food so seriously to the point where you feel anxious to eat anything.

When you start feeling like that, it's time to step back and make sure that your newfound love for the gym isn't turning into an obsession. That will be very bad for your health, as you'll end up ignoring other important areas for you to focus on -- like your mental health. When you're under too much stress, you definitely can tell a difference in your attitude.

Going back to food for a minute, I have to admit that one of the top mistakes I see with newbies to the world of low carb world is that they try to demonize protein. The truth is that protein has a lot of different purposes in the body.

Did you know that your skin is technically made from mostly protein, as well as your hair? Did you also know that the body uses protein every day to handle the connections between enzymes, as well as hormones, neurotransmitters,

DNA pairs, and everything in between.

We're always using up protein, so we need new protein taken in everyday for the body to turn it into different fuels depending on the purpose. All of these exchanges take place without your interaction or even your consent. Pretty neat, eh? Aside from the lack of control part, of course. (20)

If you're used to a high carb, low fat diet, most of your calories will come from carbs rather than protein. In a high fat, low carb style way of eating, you'll get a lot of your calories from fat as well as from protein.

If you can pair the two in terms of a good steak, that's even better. What you need to do is incorporate plenty of protein, but you can get it from more than one source. There's no need to try to get everything from just beef or chicken or whatever.

You can do whatever would be easiest in terms of your compliance. If you mix up protein sources, the chances of you staying with your way of eating will actually stick. Of course, your coworkers might get tired of you having good leftovers to take in to work with you.

There are some sources of plant protein that you can turn to as well that are still within the low carb spectrum of people. You can go with soy as well as textured vegetable protein, but some people have problems with soy. (21)

I like to have a good hearty breakfast now with plenty of meat and eggs. That seems to handle my protein requirements just fine. I can also get fish, chicken, lamb, goat, turkey, duck... it's completely up to you to figure out what proteins you like the best.

There's nothing like a great workout and having wonderful low carb food afterward. That alone should be enough to help you stay as compliant as possible.

Make sure that you're looking at calculating your own protein requirements. You will need to take your current lean body mass and multiply that by 0.8 grams. For someone that's lightly working out, this is fine. (22) If you're someone that weighs 200 pounds, this means that you're going to require 160 grams of protein a day.

Before you freak out like I did at the beginning, realize that you can go with some shakes and other ways to sneak in a bit more protein. As time passes, you'll want to use real food rather than shakes, which is the way it should be.

Is it possible to get too much protein? Some experts, such as Dr. Gail Butterfield, PhD, RD, indicate that too much protein can definitely be a bad thing, as it can stress your kidneys out, triggering dehydration issues. (23)

However, my personal experience says that "too much" is far too subjective to necessarily define what "too much" protein would honestly be across the board. You might want to play with the numbers in real time until you find a protein variable every day that helps you with whatever your fitness goals are.

Protein is very filling, and you might be surprised to find that it could take you a lot more time to handle lunch for everyone. You can always go easy on the protein until you get used to thinking in terms of low carb. Don't forget to enjoy your protein with healthy fats like coconut oil and ghee. This will contribute to the sense of feeling full without bursting at the seams.

Although I tackled a big topic today, there are still plenty of other issues to cover in the "mistakes..." series.

7 ALCOHOL & CARBOHYDRATES

Today's topic is one that I want to sink my teeth into right away, because it's one that constantly comes up in the world of low carb: is alcohol really something that can derail your weight loss plans? The answer is clear, but it tends to make people upset: absolutely.

Alcohol is definitely a factor, and it's one that you're going to have to manage as soon as possible. That's not to say that all alcohol is bad. I feel that if you want to indulge and enjoy a few drinks, you should definitely do that. But you have to be able to deal with the consequences.

Some drinks, such as Sangria, can have as much as 12g of carbs in a single glass. This means that if you throw back 8 of these drinks, you're looking at almost 100g. This might have been okay in your high carb days but 100g is awfully high for low carb lifestyle eating, and many seasoned low carbers stay well under that range.

The best thing that you can do is start learning what would be the best alcoholic beverages for your low carb lifestyle. A sweet dessert wine is going to have a lot more carbs than a dry wine, and a liqueur may have plenty of sugar dumped into it as well. (24) So your best bet for drinking would have to be with distilled spirits.

That's where you're going to have just the alcohol that you would like to drink. These are all zero carb, or very close to zero carbs served. (25) Yet it's the mixers that can still get you in trouble.

Margarita mix can be as high as 30 grams of carbohydrates. So if you're only on a 60g a day allotment for your lifestyle plan, you might find yourself a little crunched for space to enjoy anything else. In that case, 30g takes up half of your "points" for the day.

Beer tends to be fairly high carb unless you see signs for low carb beer. However, many drinking aficionados comment that the selections for truly "low carb" beers is very lacking. Your mileage, of course will vary.

I can't say that I drink a lot, as the urge to drink just doesn't occur to me. If you want to enjoy a few cold ones on the porch while you wait for the sun to go down, that's fine.

But you have to make sure that you're accounting for everything that you eat and drink in order to get the best results out of your new lifestyle. That's the big mistake that people make with alcohol. They simply assume that it's not going to affect them at all. Then when the scale doesn't move forward, there are a lot of hurt feelings.

The truth is that there are a lot of things that can cause problems with losing weight. You may not be moving the scale, but you may be getting tighter measurements than you expected.

At the very beginning of my low carb journey, I found myself getting frustrated that the scale didn't move as fast as I thought it should be moving, but I was surprised to see that my measurements had gotten tighter since I moved back. There are just times when you have to realize the scale is going to lie to you and make you frustrated. Don't give in to those moments!

The bigger question here is whether or not alcohol can

really hurt your weight loss chances. Technically speaking, alcohol is considered a poison to the body, and it will cut back on other systems to free up resources to clear the alcohol out of your body. This is part of the reason why you feel so bad after drinking. (26)

If you are going to drink, limiting yourself to a moderate dose will not only keep you from the heavier side effects of heavy drinking or binge drinking, while still letting you feel like you can socialize with anyone.

If you're just starting out in life, you might feel like you're the only person for miles that is playing by the book, but the reality is that everyone will eventually be bound to the same rules. They can't really outrun biology on this one. No matter what happened to them, don't get caught up in their background drama.

This little series is definitely taking off. Everyone has sent in such kind letters, notes, and recommendations, and I want to try to incorporate them all into the series.

8 UNDERESTIMATING CARBS

Whether you're on the go or staying at home, one thing is clear; carbs matter. I definitely had to learn this the hard way, and it's not a mistake that I'm fond of really sharing with all of you.

But that's the only way that we ever learn in life and I hope that my misadventures in low carb lifestyle eating will serve as examples of what to avoid completely.

Today's mistake is simple: most newcomers to the world of low carb assume that anything that is low carb is fair game, as "calories don't matter".

The truth is that caloric intake definitely does matter, as calories are representatives of the energy within food you eat. Some foods will be much more nutrient dense and have more calories. Other foods will not be as nutrient dense. It's up to you to use a good nutritional count resource to keep track of things like this (27).

Carb intake matters as well. Just because you think everything you're eating is low carb doesn't mean that it is. Sure, one serving is well under the low carb banner, but what happens when you learn that the "serving size" on your plate matches 4 of the servings on the package? That's a little disconcerting, to say the least. When I was trying out low carb for the first trial run, I felt like I would never succeed at this lifestyle change. I had plenty of friends telling me to just skip it, it was too hard to be low carb.

Well I'm not the type of person that just sits and gives up before things have really gotten off the ground. I wanted to give low carb living an honest chance, giving myself room to turn it into a lifestyle. My low carb mentor was a guy that had totally transformed himself with low carb eating, and I wanted to follow in his footsteps.

He admitted to me personally that things weren't always easy during his transition, but he doesn't even have cravings anymore. Even though I conditioned myself a little playing soccer, I still found myself with cravings for things I knew I shouldn't be eating.

Low carb will relieve a lot of that, especially if you go into ketosis. It's a state where the body burns ketones (fat) for fuel rather than glucose. There is a small amount maintained by the body for areas where glucose is still heavy, but for the most part -- ketosis is about burning fat for fuel, not sugar (glucose)

Do you know how many carbs you want to start with before you start tweaking your diet? Dr. Atkins made famous the "Induction" phase of his popular low carb plan. This induction phase is designed to get you moving into ketosis and enjoying some early weight loss.

Sometimes when we want to make a lifestyle change, we need to see some results to convince our own minds that there's still hope out there left for us. After being burned by so many different diets I wanted something that I could commit to for a while. So I totally understand it if you're thinking the same thing.

Looking up carb counts is easy if you're going to focus with just the online side of things. Here's a resource to help you do that (28).

From here, you just need to make sure that you take the

first few weeks of your entrance into low carb slowly. Look at all of the carb counts for all of the foods that you plan to make. While this is a bit tedious in the beginning, the reality is that you're not going to have to do it forever.

While I'm on the subject of actually counting your carbs, you need to be aware that there is such a thing as net carbohydrates. All you have to do in order to figure out the true carb count is to take the total carbohydrates listed and remove any sugar alcohols or fiber from the main amount.

So if you had a food where there was 20g of carbs but there's 12g of fiber, you're only looking at 8g of net carbohydrates that would actually affect your daily total.

Sometimes that allows us to eat things that we would otherwise shy away from. The more foods that you can be open to, the less likely it is that you're going to get bored with low carb living (29).

I know I say it a thousand times in each little "guide" but the truth is that this is something that you are going to have to turn into a lifestyle. If you don't, you'll always be unhappy with what you're really doing.

Give yourself plenty of space in the beginning to make mistakes -- I know I did. Being good to yourself is the key to a great life, and I want you to have the body you've always wanted. Trust me, it's in there -- and as you follow along in this series of "mistakes", you're bound to gain the power you need to bring your dream physique to life!

9 GOING ZERO CARB

Covering all of these different low carb mistakes definitely makes me feel nostalgic! Now that low carb eating is truly my lifestyle, it feels odd to go back to a time where I really didn't know any better and I did a lot of things where I thought they would be helpful for me.

It doesn't make sense to relive all of my mistakes, but I figure if it helps at least one person truly embrace this lifestyle with open arms, then any embarrassment on my part can't be too bad, can it? Nope, not at all.

Today's mistake is simple: going zero carb, as in avoiding as many carbohydrates as possible. This is a very destructive trend within the low carb field, and it's one that doesn't seem like it's going anyway any time soon.

Some people are so mesmerized by the idea of cutting out a lot of carbs that they feel like carbs are the enemy no matter what. The truth is that an entire class of macronutrient isn't the bad guy. It's how we use that macronutrient when we're inside the house as well as when we're not at the house.

What you do determines how your health becomes. If you continue eating the same way you did before you went

25

into low carb living, you'll gain back weight like crazy. Yet there's no need to swing the pendulum in the other direction. There are some serious risks involved with a zero carb diet, including serious glucose deficiency. (30)

Glucose is used in quite a few systems, including the brain as well as the nervous system. Your body needs some carbohydrates in order to literally keep you thinking and functioning. So when you don't give your body what it's really looking for, there is going to come a point where you stop functioning optimally.

While it's true that we can synthesize glucose from protein through gluconeogenesis, the reality is that we're not going to be able to do so nearly as well as animals do (31). When you sit down and start planning your meals, you want to make sure that you're not cutting out all of your carbohydrates.

You want to still be able to enjoy starchy root vegetables like turnips and you want to also look at other great tasting whole foods. I'm very fond of big green salads -- easy clean up, and it's already wife approved. My wife likes knowing that I'm taking care of my health and not making a big mess in the kitchen at the same time. :)

There's another issue at hand with zero carb diets that doesn't get discussed as much: kidney stones. There is a study from the Journal of Child Neurology, posted in April of 2007 that explored the link between kidney stones and a ketogenic diet where very few carbohydrates are actually consumed. The link is due to the higher concentration of uric acid via protein metabolism. (32)

It makes sense to step back and look at the bigger problem: extremism. Anytime that you have to go to extremes there's going to be side effects that we haven't looked at. Excess uric acid production can lead to gout very easily, which is a very painful condition. (33)

The other issue with zero carb diets, in my opinion is simple; it's hard to stick to. Like those big green salads?

You're not going to be able to have that on a zero carb diet. Want to have berries? You're not going to be able to have fruit of any kind on a zero carb diet.

Chocolate is out too, and even heavy cream is a bit suspect -- most zero carb followers wouldn't touch that either. Meat and fat gets tiring very quickly -- even when the monotony is broken up with a single egg. It's just not going to be sustainable.

Most people that are looking into a zero carb diet want to lose weight quickly. While I complete understand that perspective very well, there is something to be said about losing weight for the right reasons and the right way.

So if you're looking at whether or not zero carb is worth it for you, take my advice -- it's really not. You can still get to a healthy weight simply by shifting your carbs down a little bit and getting some exercise in.

Sleeping better than you have in a long time will actually have more to do with your weight loss than the extreme zero carb stance you could take. Once you mess with your metabolism, you're never quite the same.

Wouldn't it just make sense to embrace a program that wouldn't make your children feel guilty because you're eating something different?

Next installment of these little "mistakes" should be a good one, albeit it a bit controversial.

10 NOT GETTING ACTIVE

Is exercise a dirty word in your book? If so, I apologize up front because this installment of the "mistake" series will have a lot of references to exercise in it. It's something that I personally feel everyone should do even if they ultimately decide that they're not going to follow a low carb lifestyle plan.

Exercise is something that can breathe new energy into us that we never knew existed. (34) For me, it's not a worry about whether it contributes directly to my weight loss. I feel better and much more committed to the obligations I have set forward for myself, which leads to a bigger, brighter day than if I avoided the exercise.

For you science buffs in the audience, exercise does have some key benefits. A report from the United Nations Inter-Agency Task Force on Sport for Development and Peace lists numerous benefits of "sport and physical activity", including the ability to prevent hip fractures, as well as increasing the overall independence of older people.

Exercise can expand lung capacity and make breathing a lot easier. (35) We need to be stimulated in life, and exercise is something that's very stimulating. There's no reason to believe that it's impossible to get started with exercise. I suspect that's why so many people profess to hate working out -- they feel like it has to be something complicated.

I disagree. If we take out the word "exercise" and put in the word "getting active", the picture begins to look a lot clearer. Getting active can mean anything from grabbing the stroller and taking baby out for a walk around the neighborhood all the way up to going for a relaxing swim with family and friends.

You don't have to feel like the gym has to be where all of the exercise comes from. If you want to avoid the gym and explore the world around you, this is perfectly fine.

When I got into low carb eating, a lot of people told me that working out wasn't necessary. I loved playing soccer and I had done it enough that I felt much more comfortable working out than just sitting around the house.

Will you lose weight without working out? Certainly. However, it's important to realize that you boost your ability to lose weight dramatically when exercise is added.

If you're fighting the blues here and there, you'll find that exercise has long been considered "Nature's Prozac" (36), due to its mood lifting effects. You don't have to work out so hard that you're a sweaty, dripping mess that hates life.You do however have to make sure that you're doing something that makes you happy. For me, that's playing soccer when I can find the time to play a few games. For others, it might be coaching a sport with their children.

You'll find that diet and exercise go hand in hand. You want to make sure that your way of eating compliments the other goals in your life. It's not just about looking good, as so many people believe.

You're making these changes because there's probably a health scare that you're facing. There are numerous diseases linked to obesity, so losing weight can do nothing but make you feel better.

There are a few warnings that I will throw in here, since

we're on the subject of exercise. You really need to make sure that you're talking with a doctor if you are already obese. You want to make sure that you lower your chances of injury as much as possible.

The doctor will also want to monitor your progress and make sure that they are being as encouraging as possible. You will need to let them know what you're eating. This is also where a food log tends to come in handy.

You can show the doctor the healthy changes that you're making. Keep in mind that not every doctor is wise about low carb lifestyle eating, so you may have to educate them.

And if I may be a little egotistical, these "mistakes" guides would be a wonderful addition to your doctor's reading library as well. They will appreciate the extensive references to great medical journals and authoritative websites. (37)

Back to the topic at hand, changing your eating life isn't enough. You're going to have to get active, but this isn't the end of the world. You just pick something you really like to do, and the rest will fall into place. Don't worry, I still have plenty of tips for you so that you avoid the classic mistakes of going low carb.

11 FOOD ALLERGIES

Are you ready for this episode? Because really, if you're trying to get into low carb, chances are good that you might run into a few food intolerances and even food allergies. I wanted to clarify what I mean by both of these terms before we get too deep.

You see, food allergies are what you imagine to be "the worst" of them all -- peanut allergies, shellfish allergies... there are even people who are allergic to bananas and strawberries. The level of the allergic reaction can go from mild to severe, where the exposure can create a situation where emergency medical attention is required. That's not a good thing at all.

Food intolerances are a bit sneakier. According to Dr. Mark Hyman, a leading expert on food intolerances, these are more the ones that subtly cause inflammation and make you feel sick over time rather than all at once.

Most people would rather have the immediate reaction and know what to stay away from than have to deal with intolerances that may not fully manifest themselves for quite a while. This means that you could have done years of damage to your body and never been aware of it. (38)

When I first heard about food intolerances, it was from a dear friend of mine. She told me that she discovered that she was gluten intolerant. Well, if you live in the States or even abroad, you'll find that most things are made from wheat. Finding substitutes to dishes can be challenge but apparently it can be done. (39)

There are a few ways to test for food intolerances. The best way to go would be to do an elimination diet where you slowly remove things one step at a time from your diet for a little while, then slowly add them back in. People have done food elimination diets in order to discover intolerances to eggs, wheat, dairy products, shellfish, and even tomatoes. (40)

The reason why you want to check for food intolerances is because new studies are out that indicate these intolerances can actually keep you away from your goal weight. If you're going to go low carb, you have to also make sure that you're screening for any intolerances that could be blocking the weight loss that you so rightly deserve.

There's no reason to give low carb living a hundred percent of your attention and then be derailed by something that you can control. It can be hard to give up foods that you really, really like --even when they are technically within the scope of low carb living. But you have to make sure that you're watching out for your overall health.

Inflammation is a "silent killer", constantly waiting in the wings to alert us to danger. The problem comes when the danger factor never stops -- we lose the power to stop triggering the inflammation, and it runs wild. (41)

Food intolerances cause weight gain through inflammation. The two are now directly linked by scientific evidence, which means that you no longer have any reason to indulge in foods that you know are contributing to bad health. I like my junk food as much as any other guy, but there comes a point where enough is truly enough.

When you want to make the remaining years of your life the best of your life, you can't just sit and hope that everything will line up. You have to know that things are going to go well because you're making a complete lifestyle change from the ground up. And yes, I know that this is easy for me to say.

All I can do is present to you the information. You are the one that still has to read everything and decide for yourself -- is this the year that I truly change my life, or am I just kidding myself? If you're just kidding yourself, then you might as well admit that. It's better to admit that you're not ready for something than to indicate that you are and still spin your proverbial wheels.

I fully believe that each and every one of you has the ability to take back control of your health. Will this year be that year? The tips here in this little mistake may help you save your own life one day. Look into not only food intolerances, but good substitutions.

Remember how we prepared for low carb living by getting rid of everything that didn't make us feel healthier, happier, and heartier? Well, you're going to have to do this for all of your food intolerances as well. Don't give up -- you have all of the power within you to conquer this, too! And I still have plenty of low carb mistakes to share with you.

12 NOT TRACKING

Before I begin today's "Mistake", let me ask you a blunt question. Are you ready?

Here it goes: are you honestly committed to being low carb at this point? You see, we're at Mistake #12 and I wanted to make sure that you're still on board with this. If there's anything you need, let me know. If you just want to vent about how frustrating this transformation process can be, I'm here for that too.

But you have to be on board, and that means doing the things asked in the very beginning. But of course, if you really don't know what's going on, then you're having to just learn along the way.

Guess what? Everyone has had to do that, when you really think about it. Even people that claim to be incredibly good at low carb now had to start from scratch at one point. You can't just hope that you'll be at the finish line from the beginning. But if you're really willing to learn, all things become possible.

Now then, let's move on to Mistake #12 officially, okay? This one is very near and dear to my heart, because I'm an attention to detail type of guy. #12 is simple: not tracking what you're eating. A lot of newbies think that they really have no need to track their food intake from day to day, week to week, and month to month. This is a big mistake on a lot of different levels.

You see, if you aren't tracking your food, you can't tell what's really affecting you and what isn't affecting you. You have no idea what's really going on. You have no way to really reach out to the rest of the low carb community. Believe me, I understand what a pain tracking can be.

When you don't have a lot of time as it is, the last thing you want to do is write down all of the food you ate. I mean that -- you need to track everything that goes into your mouth.

You need to make sure that you're tracking that sneaky shake that you had at the mall. You need to track the cake you shared with a friend "just because". You need to basically see all of the little ways throughout your day that you can sabotage your own weight loss goals.

This will lead to something amazing: the power to see exactly where you're going wrong and correcting it fast. Our memories are really short if we had to rely on them instead of notebooks, sticky notes, and computer data stored safely elsewhere.

One study that immediately comes to mind used a dietary log and found that people who stick to the plan of their choice lose more weight than people who only handle things sporadically. (42)

Does it get easier over time? Absolutely! There's another interesting study that says that tracking weight loss leads to an easier time in true maintenance, but your mileage may vary. (43

Let's not forget that if you can monitor your own food intake, you start becoming more mindful of food. Many researchers point out that the presence of food everywhere does make it harder to actually maintain a healthy weight, but that doesn't mean that it's impossible.

It just means that you're going to have to try a lot harder than you might have expected. That's all there is to it, really. Once you are committed to going low carb and staying there, you're going to love having the data to look back on. If you find that a food is triggering weight gain, you can remove it easily.

You just drop it from your list. If the problem persists, look into another food. Generally speaking, a lot of low carbers cannot go overboard on the nuts and seeds because they're so overjoyed to have a snack.

I have found that I really can't go too deep into snacking on almonds and walnuts. They are delicious nuts and very affordable all things considered, but they tend to create a craving response in me. Your mileage may vary, but that's just what I've observed.

Tracking doesn't have to be something complicated -- you just have to write it all down. There are also online sites (44), (45) that can help you with this as well.

Now is the best time to get serious about your low carb journey. Of course, I'm far from finished giving you my top mistakes I see all of the time in low carb!

13 THE ART OF PATIENCE

Apathy. Fatigue. Worry. Stress. All of these things together create a situation that's absolutely dangerous for a low carber, especially one that's new to the industry.

You'll find yourself wondering why you made this lifestyle change in the first place. Trust me, I know. When I first went low carb, I thought that I was just going to melt because there wasn't an easy navigational system through the grocery store.

There weren't people next to me to coach me on and encourage me to make better choices. I was frustrated that I couldn't just order things the way I was used to, and I was very frustrated because of that.

I wanted to do something, anything to get past this point. I wanted to figure out how to make everything fit together...but a bigger part of me wanted to give up because I wasn't seeing results.

The truth is that low carb can take a little while. Everyone's body is going to be different, and that means that you can't put yourself on a "countdown clock". Your mental health status matters when it comes to weight loss. (46)

You may end up having to change the way you're measuring your goals. If the scale isn't moving (47), then it might be a matter of looking at inches. If you've lost inches without the weight changing, your body could be adding muscle slowly but surely.

In my case, I found that tracking my progress with a tape measure was far superior to tracking by the scale. It wasn't ruled by the scales tendency to swing back and forth a pound or two depending on my activity level and water.

For women, keep in mind that your hormones are at play far more than within men. If your hormones are out of balance, you could be keeping more water, or losing fat more slowly. A woman's body fat percentage is much higher than a man's due to the fact that most women, barring medical issues, can bear children.

It's not always a pleasant thought to realize that weight loss is going to be more difficult, but think about it from a different perspective. Once you can get that weight off, you're going to feel empowered because you beat the odds.

I fully believe that with the right mindset, everything is possible. (48) If you're feeling like you're not getting the results you really want from low carb, giving up on the lifestyle change isn't the right idea. It's time to refine further, and I have a few tips on that.

First and foremost, you might want to look at your food log again. I've discussed why keeping track of your food is so important already, but if you need a refresher, it's all about accountability.

You cannot change things that you don't know about. Nobody remembers every single thing that they've eaten for the last three weeks without help.

After the food log, you need to actually see what you're eating and whether or not it's affecting you. Nuts tend to be something that low carbers love, but it can keep them from weight loss. I used to snack on nuts until I realized how many nuts were being consumed every week. That's a lot of calories consumed, and my energy requirements may not have supported this.

Your portion sizes do play a role. There's nothing wrong with keeping a set of measuring cups close by, as well as a food scale. Yes, this means that you might have to invest a little into your new lifestyle but it's better than having to pay the doctor for more medication!

That's about it for this low carb mistake episode. As always, I'm looking forward to hearing from you. If there's anything I can do to help you become healthier, more vibrant and happier, do let me know.

14 WORKED UP OVER THE SCALE

This episode is probably going to drive a few low carbers crazy, because they seem to be obsessed with the scale. It's to the point where some people check the scale five times a day to see all of the different fluctuations.

Checking your weight is important, and I don't want to tell you that it's not important. However, the idea of having to check the scale all of the time? Not good. It just doesn't make any sense!

The scale can tell you about your total weight, but most of the time it gets your body fat percentage off. There are different ways to measure body fat -- with calipers, with home scales that use bioelectrical impedance (49), or going with a DEXA scan. The DEXA scan can only be done at certain clinics and hospitals, and it's very expensive. (50)

It's time to move away from weight and look at other factors that determine our health. If you're still not sleeping at least eight hours a night in a dark room without electrical interferences, then weight should be the last thing that you should be worrying about.

On the other hand, if you're finding that your sleep is good but your food is off, then you know that you need to work on that. I talk endlessly about keeping good logs, but people still won't do it. They say that they're far too busy to think about everything that they eat. These are usually the same people that complain about being on a stall.

You have to know that a plateau isn't just when you stop losing for a week. It's usually when your weight has not moved in at least 3-4 weeks. (51) You have to be prepared to look at your current weight and see if you're already not at a weight your body is comfortable with.

The leaner you go, the more your body will hold onto the fat that it has left. This is a biological imperative to keep us alive. The body doesn't know the difference between "starvation" and "trying to get a bikini body".

I look at myself now as a man in his 30s and realize that I'm not going to get the super slim physique that I had at 19 -- it's not going to happen unless I engage in behaviors that are destructive to my body over time.

Sure, I'd like to have a lot more muscle tone, but that comes in time. There's only so far that you can take things before they become unhealthy.

So if you're going to get worked up over the scale, you're going to find that you're missing out on a lot of benefits. It shouldn't be immediately about how much the scale is telling you that you weigh.

You have to think about the amount of fat lost, which can be hard to figure out on a scale. Even if you're going to a personal trainer who can measure your bodyfat with calipers, there's room for error in that too. (52)

I think that the scale is a handy way to gather information, but it shouldn't be viewed as the end all be all of everything. You have to make sure that you're thinking about how to take care of your body for the long term.

That's what it really means go to lifestyle. You're no longer just concerned with a certain look locked to a certain weight. It's about becoming healthier and stronger over time.

Don't forget that if you're incorporating strength training into your new lifestyle, that muscle is far more dense than fat. This means that you can lose inches without losing weight. I'll definitely take looking better to having to weigh a certain amount, wouldn't you? Hang in there -- the next episode is right around the corner.

15 IGNORING HORMONAL FUNCTION

Think hormones only apply to women? Think again! The human body is literally ruled by hormones, and you have to make sure that they are in sync with each other. This is a tall order, because stress can affect hormonal balance in both men and women. (53)

One of the big mistakes made with low carb as a lifestyle is ignoring hormonal function. This little episode is designed to get you in the loop about it so you can continue to make better decisions for your health.

Did you know that cholesterol is a major player in terms of hormonal function? Your body has to synthesize hormones from cholesterol. (54) That's why low cholesterol diets aren't as healthy as you might think.

Vitamin D is also derived from cholesterol production. So you have to make sure that your diet contains a good amount of cholesterol or your hormones are already going to be in trouble. This is the problem with low fat diets in a nutshell. (55)

You'll find an abundance of healthy fats from low carb, which means that your hormonal levels should automatically balance out without too much intervention and interference from you. It's all part of the plan to change the body naturally. After you do that, everything else will be fairly straightforward in life. You'll start picking up better health naturally as long as your low carb diet is set up properly.

What I mean by this is that you want to avoid making the mistakes I did. I ignored hormonal function and I still feared fat because of what I read. Saturated fat actually isn't a bad thing in the world of low carb dieting. (4) It's a protective measure against heart disease, not a cause of heart disease.

This is a big step for a lot of people to grasp, because we've been taught by so many sources that saturated fat is really the devil here. It's actually not the case, and that means that the steak with all of the fat on it is really a blessing, not a curse!

There are other hormones at play as well. Insulin is a major hormone that controls blood sugar, while leptin and ghrelin work together to handle hunger. Think that's the end of the hunger issue?

Not at all -- there's also cholecystokinin, otherwise known as CCK. This is a hormone that signals to the body when it's time to digest fat and protein, and it can also suppress hunger as well.

You need to have leptin because it tells the body basically when it's full. High levels of leptin lead to resistance (56), which makes it harder for you to lose weight overall. If you have a significant amount of weight to lose, your problem actually pay be leptin resistance.

You have to fix that through being conscious of when you're eating, as well as what you're eating. Grains are a major problem when it comes to leptin resistance, so it makes sense to get those grains out of your diet.

The best part? Low carb takes care of this for us, so we don't really have to think about it. Most grains are going to be high carb anyway.

Monitoring yourself via your food log is a good way to make sure that you're already getting the hormone altering effects of low carb out of the way on your end.

I'm a big believer in the idea that if you're already doing everything you can, there's nothing else for you to do. You just need to trust the process and keep low carbing. I wish you the best of luck with your low carb lifestyle. Next episode will be right around the corner.

16 IMPORTANCE OF FAT

Fat on low carb isn't just a good thing -- it's a great thing. The more fat that you can add to your low carb diet, the fuller you will be and the more stable you will become. Dietary fat isn't just for our general health -- it affects so much more. One of the top mistakes I see in low carb from newcomers is a fear of fat.

It's easy to see where the fatphobia comes from, and I'm not trying to make fun of anyone. Most people have been brought up in a culture that praises high carb, low fat, as well as encouraging people to strip out as much fat as possible. If you go to convenience stores and supermarkets, you're not seeing full-fat items -- you're seeing low-fat, "healthy" items. Dietary fat isn't linked to excess weight gain at all (57)

There are numerous vitamins that are only fat-soluble, and that means that you have to have fat to absorb them properly. We've covered good fats before (2), but it's time to revisit why they are so good for us. Going with oils that have minimal processing is a good thing. Animal fats can be high in saturated fat, a protective measure that lowers your risk of heart disease. Great sources of fat include:

- **Coconut oil**: contains lauric acid, which can increase good HDL cholesterol. In addition, coconut oil can help the body raise its stores of pregnenolone, which is a substance that helps us form many of the other hormones needed by the body. (58)
- **Tallow**: heat stable while cooking, and very delicious beef fat.
- **Avocado**: packed with healthy fat, potassium, fiber, B-vitamins...what's not to love about avocado? (59)
- **Butter**: a healthy fat that contains not only conjugated linoleic acids, which are believed to prevent cancer, but it also contains butyric acid, an essential fatty acid that can aid in treating depression. (60)

Now, when I tell people about the joys of fat, they assume that it has to be eaten with a spoon like ice cream. That's absolutely not what I'm saying here. I'm saying that you need to incorporate fat into your life the way you would have before going low carb.

If you're going to fry something on the stove, reach for the coconut oil instead of the vegetable oil that's probably already rancid. If you're going to bake, there's nothing wrong with brushing the baking dish with coconut oil.

It's very heat stable and won't break down like other fats. If you're hungry for a snack, an avocado with salt and pepper could be much more filling than yet another sugary sweet treat that's going to just leave you hungry in a few hours.

If you can handle dairy, you'll find that heavy whipping cream is a great source of fat. You can even add heavy whipping cream to your coffee. In fact, you might get so used to having this cream in your coffee that you won't want to have pesky sugar clogging up the flavor pipes. You just have to test things out, see what really works for you.

If you're a big meat eater, you'll find that adding fat is

easy. You can use the coconut oil to cook with, but don't forget to top your meat with butter. At first, it might sound weird but it's actually very delicious.

I love adding a bit of butter to my rib eye steaks, as I feel like I get the best of both worlds. Don't ignore the meat on the bone, as you can save the bones and turn them into a good stock or a hearty broth that will heal you while you're sick.

I have yet another episode coming up -- are you ready? This next one is going to be VERY important...

17 IGNORING SUPPLEMENTATION

One of the largest mistakes you can make as a low carber is assuming that all traditional medicine is bad for you. On a simpler level, this comes into play when supplementation is mentioned. A lot of low carb newbies feel that low carb is the answer to all of their prayers, so they skip over the things that the doctor tells them.

Folks, I have bad news for you: you're still going to have to see a doctor, and you're still going to have to make sure that you're talking to them about your health. Not only that, but when the doctor says that you need to supplement, you need to get with the program.

Supplementation is actually a big deal because you're addressing deficiencies in the body. I am not saying that low carb hasn't changed my life, but you never really realize just how much a lifestyle change can affect you until you get sick. I wasn't sick in terms of being able to handle the rest of my life, but I was someone that needed to get deficiencies handled.

As a low carb newbie, you're probably not in balance already. That means that hoping to get everything from food is just torture. It's better to seek out resources that can make the journey easier. If you are low on Vitamin D, you might not get as much as you need from the sun in order to start feeling better. (61) What's worse is that if you are a fairly tan person, you might not be absorbing as much Vitamin D as someone with fairer skin (62)

Vitamin D is not the only supplement that you'll need as you enter your low carb lifestyle. I've found that magnesium carries strong benefits for me, and I will assume that you can benefit from it as well. Magnesium is used by the body in a wide variety of processes, including energy production, muscle relaxation, and cholesterol adjustment.

If you don't have enough magnesium, your body will not be able to handle these processes adequately. This is why people feel tired and fatigued far more than they would like -- their body simply doesn't have what it needs to function optimally. There is a world of difference between living and thriving, between just getting through your days and being able to thrive. If you want to thrive, you need to observe what you're really lacking and seeing about getting more of it into your diet, as well as additional supplements. (63)

At first, you might feel like it's unnecessary to really embrace all of this supplementation. However, the truth is that we cannot expect to get everything from a compromised food supply.

The minerals in the soil aren't at the same level as they were before, and this means that crops just aren't going to produce the same type of rich produce that was designed to nourish us from the beginning. (64)

Starting with just Vitamin D and magnesium can do wonders. I recommend looking into the role of supplementation on your own. This is something that's very subjective, as everyone is different and has different deficiencies. I'm looking forward to another episode with you, and I have another one right around the corner. Won't you join me again?

18 NOT GETTING BLOODWORK DONE

Trying to do it all on your own, low carbers? Believe me, I was in your shoes at one point. It was mostly because I was new and I was so convinced that everyone was trying to lead me away from the right path.

I was so worried that people were trying to poison my success. I was terrified that I was missing out on some grand secret that every other low carber knew but I didn't.

If you are feeling that way right now, go ahead and smile – you're truly not alone! Now that low carb is more or less my lifestyle, I don't get worked up like that. I don't feel the need to worry about how I'm doing compared to other people.

Once you know what your goals are, it's hard to really feel any type of jealousy when you see someone ahead of you. I have to remember that just as I envy the low carber that's been that way for 7 years, chances are good that I have someone new that's looking up to me. Being a role model is great, but there is some pressure to get things right.

Moving into the topic for today's episode, the top mistake that low carbers make would be to assume that they don't need blood work done, and they certainly don't have to go to a doctor.

While there is a group within the world of low carb that seems to eschew doctors, most LC'ers aren't making that choice. They're saying that while they do want to take their health back into their own hands, they don't want to get rid of the doctor, either.

Your doctor can order bloodwork for you, and also sit down and interpret the numbers. (65) Keep in mind that you still need to have a good idea of what the test should represent. While you can trust your doctor, you still need to make sure that you have your own understanding because it's your body.

So, that being said, what should you really get done? There are a few things that you want to test, including getting your complete blood cell count, which can determine whether or not you are anemic. Anemia is no joke, and it can affect men just as much as it affects women, if not more. (66)

You also want to get your Hemoglobin A1C levels checked, as this is a snapshot of your blood sugar over the last three months rather than the one you do at home with the last hour or two.

You're better off adding this bloodwork test to your list, because it can show you whether or not you've become diabetic. Diabetes left unchecked can lead to serious problems, so it's best to make absolutely sure that you're sidestepping this key issue. (67)

Getting your testosterone levels checked is very important, as testosterone has a lot of function in the male body. When men start feeling like they're beginning to lose energy and drive, a low testosterone level could be to blame for it. (68)

While it's true that you probably don't like needles and probably despise having your blood drawn, you really do need to make sure that you're going to be making that appoint with your doctor anyway. It's better to have an accurate picture of what's going on with your body rather than just assuming that your low carb diet takes care of everything.

A song as you remain calm and collected about your low carb diet, everything should be just fine. Next episode coming up soon -- so far, so good right?

19 COMPARING YOURSELF TO OTHERS

There's a terrible diseases that affects low carbers -- perhaps you've heard of it. It's not limited to newcomers, but newcomers seem to suffer from this the most. What's that disease, you're wondering? It's easy: the disease of comparing yourself to others.

What a coincidence, as this topic is the subject of our current episode. The truth is that while you might feel like you should be comparing yourself to any and every low carber that you find, that's really not what you want to do.

You really need to be thinking about how your low carb journey is going. Are you staying on plan? Are you keeping a food log? Are you exploring other forms of exercise that keep you moving? Are you talking to someone about any mental health issues that are on your mind? Do you have an outlet for your stress? (69)

All of these questions are far more interesting than worrying about what dress size someone else is wearing. You have to be comfortable in your own skin, otherwise you will just lose the weight and find that you still don't like yourself.

The truth is that even men have image issues. I will admit that I would love to go back in time and have the same body that I had when I was 19. Is that going to happen?

Probably not. Do UI really, really want that to happen? Sometimes, I do. However, now that I'm in my 30s life is so much more fulfilling. I'm married to someone that I love, and she loves me back. What more could you want?

Comparing yourself to others just sets the scene to tear yourself part for every mistake. You start wishing that you could be as on plan and strict as Mary, even though your "off plan" cheats aren't too bad. You need to make sure that you're going back to study your goals. Do you have a weight loss vision board?

You might want to stop and read it all over again. Sometimes knowing what we're working so hard for can make sure that we stay on track even when we want to fall apart. Avoiding emotional meeting is very important here. You don't want to get dragged back when you've done so much to move forward, right? (70)

Again, I'm not talking about things that I've never experienced. I've experienced it in the soccer world, where I wanted to play better than a midfielder that I admired. I had to deal with it in school, where so many students were ahead of me.

That didn't mean that I was a bad student, and I wasn't a bad soccer player either. The trouble is that I thought I had to be the #1 person all of the time. That's a bad idea because it puts a target on your back. It causes you to second guess yourself and feel like everything you do is going to blow up in your face.

What I've found is that when I start comparing myself to other people, I stop and look at everything I've achieved. This is why you need to be taking before and during photos. The afternoons can wait. Being able to look at old pictures and see how far you have come is definitely a great thing. (71)

I'm just asking you to give yourself a chance. There are numerous reasons to hang in there. Accountability can help you focus on a job well done. I'll be your accountability partner, if you let me! For now, that's it for this episode.

20 GOING OVERBOARD ON PACKAGED FOODS

This episode might be a little controversial, but I felt I wouldn't be doing newcomers any favors by hiding from the truth. Packaged foods on low carb are often seen as a godsend -- now we can be just like everyone else.

The truth is that now that I'm successfully enjoying a low carb lifestyle, I don't want to be like everyone else. I don't want to go back to my old lifestyle. I don't want to go back to feeling tired, sick, and carrying around excess weight. So if you care about having the same food as everyone else -- more power to you, but I am not in that camp.

The truth is that processed food just isn't good for us, in any way, shape or form. It's a matter of convenience, but it's one that we pay for through having more sodium than we would like, more fat that we may not be able to use as well as fats from whole foods, and a variety of other issues (72)

What you're going to have to do is figure out what type of low carber you want to actually be. While it takes more time to prepare real food, the benefits cannot be beat. You'll actually get to a point where you really don't want to deal with processed food because it doesn't taste good. We pay a lot for food that has a uniform taste -- all of those extra preservatives have to go somewhere, and that "somewhere" is your body.

A lot of the times where people talk about a plateau on low carb, they're being blocked by processed food. They don't want to admit that because then their convenience factor would go away. But processed food can also have MSG, which has a variety of issue attached to it as well (73).

What you have to do is make sure that you're thinking about cooking for yourself. It's really not as hard as you think to cook low carb. There are plenty of recipes out there, along with videos. You never know -- you might get so excited about cooking that you teach someone else.

There's something about cooking that has always captured my attention. The truth is that time is really a democratic thing -- we all get the same amount of time.

No matter how you cut it, you have to figure out how to make the most of your time. Just saying that you have no time to prepare anything is really an excuse. You're better off making sure that you're taking care of your health.

The truth is that without health, we have nothing. I'm not saying that the packaged foods aren't good -- compared to high carb living, the packaged foods are a modest compromise. But you're going to be a lot better off with fresh, whole food.

Do the best you can, because low carb isn't about elitism at all. You never know -- you might start with a few convenience foods, and then move up to higher quality food. That's the best way to ensure that you've got things under control. (74)

The time is right to take this seriously. We're halfway through our episodes, and I want to take time right here, right now to thank you very much for tuning in. Deep down, my highest passion is helping you succeed. So if there's something I've overlooked or missed, please point it out to me and I'll get it corrected.

Aside from that, let me know how you're doing. Low carb is hard without support, but don't worry -- I am here for you, always! Ready for the next episode? It's coming up next!

21 NOT GOING GLUTEN-FREE

This one is controversial, but if you've already gotten halfway through our little series of episodes, you know that I'm not afraid to tackle the tough subjects. The truth that you need to hear right here, right now is that going gluten-free on your low carb eating plan is probably one of the best things that you can do.

You see, I did it more or less as a test to see how it would affect me, only to find that I want to make it part of my permanent lifestyle change. Yet if you're really just getting started, you might not realize what gluten is, why it's everywhere, or what it's really doing to your body.

You might have heard about celiac disease, a violent disease that literally attacks the body's digestive system and other connected systems. It's a miserable condition that requires strict adherence to a gluten-free diet. However, there's a new category rising: non-celiac wheat sensitivity (75), and more and more people are reporting about it.

This really isn't surprising when you look at the fact that wheat -- gluten is the primary protein of wheat -- has changed dramatically over the last few years. (76) It's designed more for high yield rather than health, and that's a big problem that's lead to a lot of other issues people have.

Are you constantly fatigued? Ready to just go back to bed? You could have an underlying gluten sensitive and not even realize it. Doing a food elimination diet (77) can help you with that, but you're going to have to be absolutely honest with yourself. Don't just read this and say "Oh, I'm not bothered by gluten, so all of the cupcakes are still fine by me!"

Hey, I'm a guy that likes to eat plenty of sweets, and I've had to cut back. If you're going low carb, you'll find that most of your wheat products are way too high carb to be eaten normally.

And even if you're going to have a tiny portion to stay within your carb range, what's the point when it's not good for you? What's the point when there are so many better choices out there?

Don't get caught up in the hysteria over wheat. It's something that doesn't really belong in your low carb meal plan anyway, and it's just going to end up making you sick. Even if you don't have symptoms of wheat problems now, what's stopping you from having problems with wheat in the future?

What's stopping you from having issues with the proteins within wheat? Even if you don't have a problem with gluten, there are other nutrient-draining properties found within wheat that should be avoided.

These are called lectins, and they can bind precious nutrients that the body needs, causing a wide variety of problems. Inflammation and wheat are connected together as well. If you followed the earlier episodes, you know that inflammation is considered the "silent killer", and lowering inflammation should be one of our top goals. (78)

The next episode is coming up! After all, your continued glowing health is my top priority. I love keeping you informed! :)

22 ROLE OF TESTOSTERONE

Think this is just an article for men? Incorrect! The truth is that both sexes produce testosterone, just at different amounts, and for different reasons. If you're going to turn low carb into a lifestyle, you have to be aware of your hormones.

I know that I talked a bit about hormones in a previous episode, but then I thought...what's the top hormones that I really wanted to highlight for these awesome people? I had to start with testosterone.

Testosterone in men is pretty important, and there are many studies that indicate just how vital this hormone really is. Testosterone is behind a man's deeper voice, his muscle mass (and ability to put on more muscle than women), and his strong bone density (79).

Low testosterone is a problem that's growing in today's modern culture, for a variety of reasons. Stress, bad diets, the environment... the list goes on and on. If you're going to get deep into a low carb lifestyle, you need to make sure that your hormonal health is going to be taken care of properly.

Are there tests for low testosterone? Absolutely. (80)

Your doctor can do a blood test to check for testosterone in the body. If you have low testosterone -- measured as less than 300 ng/dL (nanograms per deciliter) -- then it's time to look into treatment for it.

Your doctor can explore testosterone injections, which are just given every couple of weeks or so. For the men out there trying to start a family, low testosterone can put your dreams on hold. That's not something I'd want to live with, do you?

Most doctors will not connect your diet back to your hormonal health, but low carb is definitely the way to go if you're trying to watch your overall health. The reason why is easy: fat helps hormone production in both men and women, and this includes testosterone. (81)

There are plenty of great sources for fat when it comes to low carb -- butter, ghee, coconut oil, lard, tallow, duck fat... the list goes on and on. Adding these to your diet will increase your cholesterol intake, which in turn should help raise your testosterone levels naturally. Eggs are also a great source of fat as well as a host of other nutrients.

Don't just sit on the problem, hoping that things will get better. If your levels of T are too low, you might find that you're going to have to solicit a doctor's help to get things moving forward. You don't have to just ache without cause when there are so many solutions to help you out.

Ignoring the problem will only make it worse, and the side effects of low testosterone are pretty rough. They include fatigue, low libido, possible bone density loss, lowered sperm count, increased breast size... do I need to go on, or will you get yourself checked out?

As always, I am deeply concerned about your health and success on a true low carb lifestyle. Ladies, don't think I left you out -- the next episode is all about you!

23 IGNORING ESTROGEN (WOMEN)

Women's hormone health is actually such a lengthy topic, I'll be dividing it into two parts. Although I'm not a woman, I'm deeply devoted to my wife and know that helping her achieve proper hormonal health and balance is a win-win for both of us. I don't like seeing her hurt, and I want her to be as healthy as possible so we can have a long life together.

Going low carb is honestly the best way to balance the body, as you're going to be removing many toxins that hide in processed food. This is a good thing, but a deeper discussion of hormones is still required. The big hormone of note would have to be estrogen, which is produced by the ovaries. (82)

Hormone imbalance affects a great deal of women today, as environmental factors and stress set in. Simply put, it's hard for women to be in balance when so many environmental factors exist to throw her body out of balance. Pollution, toxins, heavy metals all add stress on the body, which in turn affects the mind. Even if the physical side of things is addressed, the mental health side usually isn't. Women struggle to make sense of a world that has far too many demands on them.

Addressing hormonal health means looking at levels of estrogen in the body. This has to be done at a very specific time in a woman's cycle, as her estrogen levels change dramatically depending on when the test is taken. (83)

Estrogen and progesterone work together, but both have to also be regulated by cholesterol. See how cholesterol seems to dominate the conversation when it comes to talking about hormones? Indeed, the National Institute of Health has weighed in on the discussion and found that a woman's natural levels of cholesterol will change based on which phase of her cycle she's actually in. And you thought science wasn't interesting? (84)

These data points imply something a bit more important and often overlooked -- that low fat diets just don't work. I fully believe that low carb is incredibly nourishing to both men and women, but women seem to fare even better on low carb than men do. To me, this highlights the dangers of low fat diets more than anything else.

Yet you don't have to just take my word for it. If you want to really see the difference in your own life in terms of taking care of your hormones, really stick to a low carb diet as a lifestyle. Get rid of all of the unhealthy seed oils and other highly processed things. This will open the door to a lot of healthy fat, including the saturated kind that so many felt was off limits before. Jump into it wholeheartedly by avoiding inflammation-spiking grains, as they tend to boost your carb level without giving you any type of nutrient satisfaction.

It can be seen as a long and complicated journey, or one of the best things that you've ever done. There is hormone treatment available for hormonal imbalance. Your doctor can follow up with you on that, if natural methods (diet, sleep, stress management) haven't taken care of the problem. Don't worry; we still have plenty of episodes left.

24 CHRONIC CARDIO

Make no mistake about it: every episode is designed to move you forward a little bit more at a time. The more I can give you in terms of information, the more likely it is that you can have a great chance at a healthy life from the inside out. That's what I'm here for, at least.

All of these things I try to pull from my experience. Where I can't do that, I pull from the direct experience of my friends and family that have made this life changing decision. The more that you can do to change your lifestyle, the healthier you will be in the long run. If you want decades to spend with the people that matter most to you, then I definitely encourage you to continue staying tuned to these episodes, and even going back to look at the other ones you might have missed.

Today's issue is all about chronic cardio. It's something that tends to pull in newcomers to the low carb lifestyle because they assume that more cardio is better. Some of it might extend from those late night television infomercials that I've heard are pretty popular, where it's all about cardio and nothing about strength training.

The science, however, is pretty clear on the role of

cardio. I'm not trying to say that cardio on its face is a bad thing, merely that you want to mix it and not spend hours doing cardio work. That's not going to help you reach for health. Remember our good buddy cortisol, the stress hormone? When we overwork our bodies, cortisol kicks in, making fat loss very difficult. (85)

My favorite study has to come out of McMaster University, where two groups were compared. The first group was all about high intensity interval training -- short bursts of very rapid activity. The other group was all about long doses of cardio -- up to 2 hours at a time. The study showed that over time, both groups improved on a similar baseline. This means that you don't have to flat out kill yourself to get into the best shape of your life. (86)

Another study (87) indicates that long distance running may contribute to poor heart health, which is something that definitely should alarm you.

The thing is, strength training doesn't have to be hardcore, aggressive, and draining. You can also mix in fun cardio things, like yoga and Pilates. Some people like Tai chi. The important thing here is that you keep moving, because being sedentary isn't where you want to be.

Trying to get more low carb is a good thing, but you also want to make sure that if you are going to start exercising heavier, that you take the time to actually adjust your food intake. You'll need the extra nutrients in order to get through your workouts. And if things get a little too tough, there's nothing wrong with stepping back.

Chronic cardio is not something that has to take over your life, when there are so many other options. Even though you might be new to the low carb lifestyle, your commitment to being healthy is what counts. Don't do anything that you aren't comfortable with, because that's just going to end in disaster. Good luck!

25 IGNORING POTASSIUM

There are some episodes that might not seem necessary until you really think about them. This is one of them. Even though you might already be deep into a low carb lifestyle, there are some essential nutrients that deserve their own space for discussion. Potassium is one of those minerals, on a wide variety of levels.

Have you ever had crippling muscle pains that you wish you could explain away? If so, you might have a problem with potassium levels. Of course, one of the go-to staples when someone mentions potassium would be a banana. Did you know that you have more choices than that on a low carb diet? Besides, bananas are extremely high carb and should be avoided, especially when you're trying to maintain healthy blood sugar. (88)

Better sources for potassium rich, low carb foods abound. You can actually go with yogurt, which averages about 380mg. Not bad, when you consider that we need about 4700mg every day in order to keep our potassium levels proper. You can also go with a cup of sweet red peppers, or a cup of Swiss chard. If you're already including these foods into your normal diet on low carb, then you're cutting down on your chances to have problems with potassium in the first place. (89)

Trust me, potassium deficiency is nothing to play with. The symptoms can include constipation, painful leg cramping, and vomiting at more severe levels. This isn't the only mineral that you need by far, but it's one of the most important. (90) Of course, I'm getting a touch ahead of myself. Potassium has a heavy role in the body that should be addressed. Potassium is considered an essential mineral because it has to regulate all of the fluids in your body. Blood pressure out of control? Your potassium levels can definitely play a role in this.

If you're having problems making your muscles contract, potassium is part of the solution to this problem. Waste removal might not be something that we really want to talk about in polite company, but potassium plays a role in this as well. You definitely need potassium, and there's no way to get around this. (91)

Keep in mind that most of the sources of potassium will not pay off until you've reached a full cup worth of the food in question. So in the case of yogurt, you're going to want to get at least a cup in. If this is a problem, you can split up the cup over a few snacks during the day. In the case of Swiss chard, you can add it to a big salad, or a big casserole. Just because you're going low carb doesn't mean that you suddenly lack for options.

It's all about getting the right amount of basic minerals that the body cannot live without. Low potassium is something that can really cause a lot of discomfort so you really want to make sure that you're looking to get this problem tended to as soon as possible. Who said that bananas and potatoes were the only sources of potassium? Just take a look around your local produce section -- you might be surprised at how many sources of potassium you'll find. I'm not quite done talking about minerals, as you'll note from the next episode!

26 MAGNESIUM

As mentioned in last episode, I really wanted to take the time to highlight some awesome minerals that the body has to use each and every day. Your body is really a series of processes that work seamlessly...until we refuse to give it something that it really needs. That's when we end up getting into a lot of symptoms and problems that tend to plague the body.

If you're going low carb and you're feeling less than top notch, mineral imbalances could be stealing your joy. I don't want that for you, which is why I started getting into the science a bit -- but always in a format that's easy to understand. These studies can be a little confusing, but that's what I'm here for -- helping you every step of the way, of course.

So, let's dig into the issue a little bit more and talk about magnesium. If you remember magnesium from chemistry class, then you already know that this mineral is on the Periodic Table of Elements. It's really that important, how cool is that? The truth is that magnesium actually helps regulate well over 300 different reactions in the body. Energy balance? Magnesium takes care of that. You actually cannot regulate your own body's metabolism without magnesium. The world around you depletes magnesium, which is why you have to make sure that you replenish your sources every single day. If you don't, then magnesium deficiency can set in. Remember our friend potassium? Well, those cramped-up muscles need magnesium just as much as they need potassium. (92), (93)

Studies have come out indicating just how vital magnesium is to the body (94), and it's important as low carbers to make sure that we get plenty of magnesium. There's no need to run out of it when there are so many great sources. Of course, if you're not interested in diet sources, you can supplement through getting Epsom salt baths. This is a very available form of magnesium that can be absorbed through the skin.

Many low carbers have found that the Epsom salt baths are a great way to manage stress, which in turn helps maintain a healthy body overall. After all, we can't survive being stressed out all the time. We can't deal with constantly being at our wit's end. I'm trying to make sure that you have as much information as possible, so that you're not stressed out as much as you might feel like you should be.

It can still be pretty overwhelming to embrace a low carb lifestyle, especially when there are so many critics towards it. You have to make sure that you're thinking carefully about your journey into low carb so that you're not tempted to just give up before you see results (as I outlined in a previous episode).

Low carb friendly sources of magnesium include avocados, green veggies, cocoa powder (as high quality as possible), salmon, mackerel, flax seed, almonds, and sunflower seeds. If you're getting a lot of protein from meat, then you'll also get magnesium from this source as well. As always, try to make sure that your protein and fat sources as of the highest quality possible. It's not necessary in the sense that you'll die without it, but going with grass-fed, pastured meats increases the bioavailability of nutrients dramatically. Plus, it's a good thing for the environment.

27 STRENGTH TRAINING

I've been looking forward to this episode, because it's one of the top mistakes that I see new low carbers getting into. They think that just diet alone will carry them through. To an extent, that's very true -- diet is a significant part of weight loss.

However, to say that exercise has no benefit is throwing the proverbial baby out with the bathwater. You need to be able to look at your options and realize that you have a way to not only achieve a lower amount of body fat, but you'll also sculpt the type of body that you really want. (95)

If you're going to get into strength training, we have to outline a few cautions that are extremely important. This is where a lot of people get discouraged by strength training, and then they don't want to really do it.

The truth is that you need to make sure that you're looking at easing into a program. If you've never done any strength training, the risk of injury is very high if you're not thinking through each and every move. This is where investing in a starter package from a qualified personal trainer is a good thing. (96)

You also want to take time learning the fundamentals of

strength training: the press, the row, the dip, the deadlift, the squat, and the pull-up. Yes, the pull-up is important when it comes to developing upper body strength. If you can't do pull-ups, don't worry -- they will indeed come in time. (97)

It might seem odd to focus on compound lifts, but there's a reason for that -- they are the most time effective way to reshape your body. Sure, you can learn a lot of isolated movements and pool them together for a longer workout, but longer is not always better.

You're going to want to be able to get your routine in, and then go do something else. Trust me, over the long run? Strength training is honestly where you want to be.

Strength training gives you a longer "boost" in metabolism, tearing through fat much better than cardio. You get a nice after burn effect that can keep you in the game longer than cardio will. I'm not saying that you have to start away with some heavy handed bodybuilder routine. That's too much even for me. Whether you're a man or woman, starting out with the basics is the key.

Some people like to start with bodyweight exercises, which can help condition before heavier weights are involved. Nothing wrong with starting out with planks, pushups, pull-ups and bodyweight squats before you graduate to actually using weights. If you ease into the world of strength training, your low carb journey can only be amplified by this, not lessened.

I'm still moving along with our episodes and the next episode ties into strength training nicely. If you're not quite ready to get with the strength training program, there's another program you can look into so that you can seriously shred fat and continue looking your best.

28 HIIT

In the last episode, I talked about how strength training is something often overlooked by the average low carb person. Yet I don't want anyone to believe that strength training is the only way to go. If you're not ready to go into strength training, or you would just like to prefer being without heavy weights, here's another angle to you to try: HIIT.

This stands for high intensity interval training, and it's not a new concept. Researchers have been measuring the effects of high intensity exercise for a long time. (98)

You'll find that HIIT brings you a host of valuable benefits, as you will not have to worry too terribly much about how to pack in a workout. Busy people will have no excuse, because the average HIIT workout is only about four minutes.

You focus on giving it your all for about one minute, then you need to take a recovery period. The commonly accepted recovery period would have to be two minutes to catch your breath, get some water, and gear up again.

This is cardio, so if you're a cardio fan, HIIT will be right up your alley. But does it really burn fat?

Absolutely. The first study that comes to mind indicates that interval training is superior to continuous training, especially when it comes to recovery periods. You will be able to recover quicker if you go with the interval training rather than the chronic cardio, where you're trapped in the gym for hours at a time (99)

There's another study that says that this is a really great exercise for women, especially if they've found that diet alone isn't reaching certain areas of the body. Keep in mind that I'm not saying that you can spot reduce your way to good health. But if strict low carb isn't helping you refine your body, adding in powerful HIIT is definitely a good fat burner (100), (101)

A few cautions. When I say intense interval training, that's exactly what I mean. You are going to be working out pretty hard, so make sure that you don't skip the basic tenets of good exercise. Proper hydration is still a must, and if you're going to supplement, I recommend keeping it simple and limited to caffeine if you must supplement at all.

Post workout nutrition will be very important when it comes to HIIT -- this is a great time to get in some protein, because the body will be looking for immediate muscle repair and replenishment.

You can get in a HIIT routine on a treadmill, or outside. This allows you to enjoy HIIT style workouts throughout the entire year. In the summer, when you get outside, you can do them around the track closest to your home.

On the other hand, if you don't have a nice track or you don't want to run on the sidewalk, you can always head to the gym. There are jump rope HIIT workouts, treadmill HIIT workouts, and HIIT workouts that just involve bodyweight movements.

You're not deprived or limited when it comes to high intensity training, and the interval format means that you can challenge yourself on your own pace, rather than being locked into someone else's progress. Don't go off of my results -- I want you to try to build your own results. I want you to try to explore HIIT on its own merits. If you're interested in the science, I've included strong references that discuss HIIT from a scientific perspective.

Remember that it's going to take you some time to get adjusted to moving that quickly. If anything doesn't feel right or you feel overly fatigued, stop immediately. I am committed to your health, but realistically I am not a doctor and this cannot be taken as medical advice.

Now then, let's move on to the next episode. In it, I tackle a mistake that's led to more than one Internet fight or two...

29 THE REAL DEAL ON FRUIT

Think that fruit isn't part of low carb? Tired of hearing low carbers say to you that you have to avoid any and all fruit or you'll gain like crazy? Think that all fruit is equal in terms of carb count and impact on blood sugar? This episode has your name all over it. Indeed, I wanted to tackle fruit because so many on low carb are mistaken about it. There's no reason why you should give up all fruit.

Fruit has a lot of benefits to it. There are some studies that point to fruit being key in reducing risk for heart disease, along with protection against certain cancers. Fruits have more than just natural sugar in them -- they have magnesium and sometimes even potassium.

Potassium is a key factor in lowering blood pressure, and magnesium works to provide energy balance throughout the body's major systems. There's no reason to skip fruit when there are so many benefits. (102)

There are low sugar fruits allowed on low carb. Personally, I love fruit and I think it's a great way to keep people compliant on a low carb lifestyle. If you try to get too extreme with cutting things out, only one thing is going to happen: you're going to go off plan. Going off plan when it comes to low carb is only going to make you miserable. The body won't know what to do with all of the carbs that rush in, leaving you sleepy, miserable, and prone to weight gaining. Why run the risk of gaining all of the weight back when you fought so hard to get it off. Keeping the weight off for life is what we're really after, when you get right down to it.

So, what fruit can you really enjoy on a low carb diet? Berries would be at the top of the list. Raspberries, blackberries, strawberries, blueberries. These are all fruits that have a high antioxidant component, which can help fight free radical production in the body. (103)

Keep in mind that the carb counts you'll find for the berries and other low sugar fruits will be based upon a serving of half of a cup. If you plan to have more berries than that, you're going to have to increase your carb count.

Depending on which plan you actually follow, this could leave you without a lot of carbs to enjoy anything else. However, if you're on a more moderate low carb plan than most, then you can definitely indulge in some fruit. (104)

Now then, my take on it may surprise you: just because I think that fruit isn't evil doesn't mean that I think you should have 6 servings of fruit every day. Fruit should be a good treat, a healthy one, but it shouldn't take the place of good dietary fats, protein, veggies, and fish. You want to have balance in your diet before you go crazy with fruit. It's been my experience that as soon as you tell people that they can have fruit, they tend to overdo it.

A lot of my low carb friends did that -- they went wild on fruit because it was a legal low carb thing, then they were sad to find out that they were gaining weight like crazy. Too much of a low carb food is still not good for you, and it can promote weight gain. That's the top thing that we want to avoid, right? Absolutely. In the next episode, we'll touch on a very powerful -- if not a little controversial -- way to lose fat on low carb.

30 KETOSIS

Ketosis is something that has a lot of fans behind it in the world of low carb, and others that feel ketosis isn't necessary at all. With so many opinions, it can be hard to figure out who is really giving you the best advice here. You need to think about the right path for you. If regular low carb is not working for you, then it might be time to turn to a ketogenic diet.

I'll warn you ahead of time -- it's definitely a lot more intense than a normal low carb diet. Some of the things that would be okay on a moderately low carb diet will not be allowed on a ketogenic one. It's a bit more "back to basics" than a lot of people are ready for. Still, the results are undeniable: you really can lose a lot of weight on ketogenic low carb. (105)

But what is ketosis, anyway? Simply put, ketosis is when the body shifts to burning fat for fuel rather than glucose for fuel. You feel less hungry, and therefore you eat less. Your body begins to burn efficiently on fat, which frees you up to burn fat rather than continue to store it. The brain, usually an organ that needs glucose, can run on what's known as ketones. Ketones are produced directly from fatty acids in the liver, and these ketone bodies are pretty efficient at powering the body (106)

The reason why ketosis and ketogenic diets get so much attention is because it's protein sparing, and therefore muscle sparing. Most restricted diets tend to strip away muscle, but not the ketogenic diet. In fact, this was a diet that was popular in the weightlifting community long before it crossed over into mainstream thinking. The good news is that you don't have to be a bodybuilder in order to reap the benefits of a ketogenic diet. (107)

There are some obvious foods to avoid, like grains of all kinds. They are far too high carb, and the more important part? You don't need them to be healthy. You will still get plenty of minerals from the veggies you eat, because those are allowed on a ketogenic diet. You want to avoid sugar in all of its pesky forms. Sugar is not only going to knock you out of ketosis almost overnight, it's a good way to put on all of those extra pounds that you worked so hard to get rid of.

Sugar and starch are sneaky, because they can hide in some of your favorite sauces. Like that house salad that they bring to you at the restaurant? Chances are good that there's sugar hiding in the dressing that's supposedly homemade. The more processed a food is, the more likely that it has hidden sugar and a ton of hidden salt that you don't need. I'm not saying that salt is evil, but at the levels that most restaurants use salt, sugar, and hidden starch? You would do better without these foods. Way better.

You can enjoy good protein, good fat, and a healthy amount of veggies without getting out of your ketogenic diet. If you really want to trial this diet, I recommend a minimum of 30 days, though I tend to prefer to tell people 90 days. You just never know what results you're missing until you check it out for yourself!

31 KIDNEY DAMAGE, KETOACIDOSIS & OTHER WORRIES

There's a few low carb myths that I wanted to address as a group today, because there are still newcomers absolutely petrified. They think that if they make low carb living part of their day to day lives, they're going to suffer terrible kidney damage, have horrible blood lipids (cholesterol), and basically shorten their lives.

The truth is that generally speaking, a low carb diet is what you make of it. If you get your veggies, meats, fats, some fish, some poultry, and some nuts and seeds -- what are you really missing out on?

Grains? They're nutritionally poor, and the only reason they have many vitamins and minerals is because they are artificially added. Do you really want to thrive on artificial vitamins, or do you want to actually thrive on real food? I know which choice I would make. (108)

People worry about whether or not their kidneys are going to be affected by a low carb diet. I'm not trying to say that you shouldn't have concerns about the diet that you choose. I'm merely saying that honestly, this is not an issue on low carb. There have been researchers from the Indiana University School of Medicine that studied low fat versus low carb, and found that there was no harmful effects brought on the body due to a low-carb diet. Even though low carb is well known for emphasizing protein, it's not going to put excess strain on your kidneys. The body is good at filtering out protein and getting it out of the body if it is in excess. (109)

Now that we've covered that, let's move on to another issue: the fear of ketoacidosis. Just like kidney damage, I don't fault anyone for getting caught up in this one. Ketoacidosis is a dangerous condition for diabetics, where high levels of ketones are found in the body, along with an inability to produce insulin. The strongest symptoms for diabetic ketoacidosis include excessive thirst, a deep need to urinate, strong abdominal pain, shortness of breath, and more. (110)

The reason why this is not an issue for low carbers is simple: low carbers still produce insulin to avoid acidosis! In other words, there is a strong difference between ketosis, which is just the production of ketones that the body uses for fuel, and ketoacidosis, a condition that affects Type 1 diabetics that need to monitor very carefully.

It can be absolutely life threatening for them. I know that I may be speaking to some Type 2 diabetics, and that's perfectly fine. Ketoacidosis is something that you probably don't need to worry about unless your pancreas is completely damaged. At that point though, you'd know and would have an insulin regimen. (111)

You can feel free to pursue a ketogenic diet if you would like to speed up your weight loss. Make sure that you are thinking about how to connect everything together for your health, of course. I wanted to dispel two of the big myths, and therefore the mistakes that low carbers get themselves into. (112) The next episode is going to be a good one!

32 NIGHTSHADES

Are you looking at refining your low carb diet? Some people are because they haven't gotten one of their goals met. For me, inflammation is a huge goal that I'm trying to focus on, because it affects long term health. Inflammation is actually a marker in most illnesses that we're all trying to avoid, including cancer, diabetes, heart disease, arthritis, and more. (113)

One word that gets thrown around in the low carb and general health communities often would be nightshades. Everyone wants to know what a nightshade is, and whether or not they should avoid it. I can't tell you with certainty whether you should avoid nightshades or not, because I have no idea what your personal history is like.

In addition, I am not a doctor, and this is definitely not medical advice, nor should it be taken that way. However, if you want to ask me friend to friend? I think that you may want to avoid nightshades if you find that you're sensitive to them, or that they don't make you feel good.

So, in a nutshell, what about those nightshades? Well, they are a plant group that is actually pretty diverse -- over 2800 species belong to the greater "nightshade" family. The scientific family is actually called Solanaceae, and the order in question would be Polemoniales. The food sin question would be potatoes, eggplant, tomatoes, sweet as well as hot peppers, pepinos, pimentos, paprika, and cayenne peppers.

The reason why some people want to avoid nightshade foods is because they have been shown to impact the way the nerves and muscles interact with each other in the body, creating painful incidents that would be best avoided if at all possible.

Indeed, a study from the Journal of Internal Academic Preventative Medicine indicates that there is some crossover between nightshades and arthritis. That's enough for me to seriously consider doing a food elimination diet, if nothing else. I'm not telling you that you automatically have to live a life without eggplant, since it's a pretty low carb dish (114).

However, you might want to remove the eggplant and the peppers to make sure that you're not sabotaging your weight loss. Remember that inflammation and weight gain are tightly linked, so anything that we can do to lower inflammation is definitely a good thing.

Make sure that you're giving your elimination diet at least a month before you add the nightshades back in. Potatoes probably won't be on the menu, since they're way too high carb, but eggplant could be added back in with no problem unless you know that you're sensitive.

Don't forget to watch out for paprika. It's a great spice that really adds flavor, but if you're sensitive to nightshades this can be a sneaky way of keeping them in without actually meaning to. The next episode will cover a serious topic that doesn't get enough attention in the low carb community. I highly recommend tuning back in.

33 ADRENAL FATIGUE

Hey, I never said that I wasn't willing to get serious when it came to giving you the best information that I possibly can. There are just some topics that might not sound like they're on topic for the low carb community, but they really are. Everyone is coming into the world of low carb with different expectations. I wasn't incredibly tired coming into this community, but I have dear friends that battle what's known as adrenal fatigue all of the time. They feel tired to the point where no amount of sleep's going to change things. Whether you call it adrenal fatigue, adrenal insufficiency, or the on-set of Addison's disease, one thing is clear: something is out of balance.

Adrenal fatigue is where the adrenals are not producing the right amount of hormones due to stress. (115). It's something that's very disputed and debated within the health community, as there's not a technical term for the mild form of adrenal insufficiency. There is however, a condition known as Addison's disease where the adrenal glands are severely damaged.

If you start searching for information on fighting adrenal fatigue, chances are good that you'll find your way into the low carb community, yet again. That's because a low carb is one of the best ways to handle adrenal fatigue. A diet that's low is sugar is unlikely to trigger heavy amounts of cortisol flooding the system. (116)

Lower carb diets are the key in making the process of fighting adrenal fatigue come together, but adherence is definitely going to be the key. Aside from diet, you have to get your stress under control. This isn't just thinking positive thoughts. As I asked my friend about how she handled her adrenal fatigue symptoms, she told me that she also had to stop exercising so much. Exercise can raise cortisol levels sky high, making it hard for the body to recover the way it normally should.

Most of the advice that you'll get online is definitely general. If you're going through signs of adrenal fatigue, the last thing that you want is to invite more stress. This means that if you've decided to add in more cardio, you might want to skip that. Taking time for sleep is going to be incredibly important.

The problem with adrenal fatigue is that most sufferers are leading highly stressed out lives. There's not enough money in the world that's going to actually replace your health. Only you can handle your health needs and that means putting yourself as a priority. (117)

I know that this one will be hard for some people, because they're always on the go. In fact, some people are just downright proud of being busy all of the time. But I know that life is what you make of it, and if you're always on the go, you never have time to really appreciate everything that's given to you.

Health is one of those things that we have to fight hard for once we lose, so it's definitely time to get things in order. If you're dealing with adrenal fatigue right now, you have my sympathies. Please look through some of the references and see if you can find some relief. All I'll say about the next episode is...it gets a little oily...

34 OMEGA-3 & OMEGA-6

Well, I said it would be oily, but you're reading the title and wondering how in the world do I get "oily" from a discussion about "omega-3 and omega-6 fatty acids"? Well, in a nutshell, these fatty acids are found in cooking oils that we know and count on. The trouble here is that the body needs a balance that modern dining culture just isn't providing.

In other words, we're getting too much of one and not of the other. Omega-3's are needed, but our diet doesn't give us enough of them most of the time. Omega-6 is the much more prevalent fatty acid chain, and it's abundant to the point our bodies are out of whack. (118)

Now, you might be thinking -- just what can I really do to increase my intake of omega-3's? It's not really that simple. In order to get the body back into balance, you need to look at the amount of omega-6 you're taking in as well.

In addition, you want to make sure that you're looking at the quality. Omega-6 fatty acids are often PUFAs, polyunsaturated fatty acids. The problem with PUFAs is that they are very fragile when you look at their chemical structure.

They degrade quickly in heat, which means them ineffective within the body. Now, you can get high quality omega-3s that don't break down like that, but you have to keep them away from heat. Not all omega-6 fatty acids are a bad thing, either -- evening primrose oil is a near godsend for women dealing with hormonal balance problems. (119)

What about cod liver oil? If you're going to supplement your low carb lifestyle with something like cold liver oil, you definitely want to make sure that it's the fermented kind.

Fermented fish oil matters because the nutrients stay intact, and the oil tends to be far more effective compared to regular cod liver oil. The bioavailability of fermented cod liver oil is incredible, and I personally recommend it to just about everyone.

I've noticed a difference in my energy levels, as well as in my hair, skin and nails. This is definitely one oil that benefits the whole body. Now, it does have an upfront cost that might be a little out of your price range but you should still check it out as soon as possible. It can really work wonders for you in conjunction with a low carb lifestyle. (120)

Do realize that oils like cod liver oil have been fermented and consumed for a very long time -- going back to the Viking era where the soldiers would simply cover the collected livers with sea water and allow nature to take its course. This is a nourishing super food of sorts that has a long, time-tested history.

The next episode is coming up, and I get to address more fun ways to get more out of your low carb lifestyle. I truly hope that you'll join me!

35 PROBIOTICS

Does low carb give you absolutely everything? That's up for debate. There are some who believe that if you're going to just commit to a low carb lifestyle, there's really nothing for you to add to it. You can just keep going through the motions, eating and enjoying life.

But I've always been one to test and tweak different things. I think that adding in probiotics is a good thing that shouldn't be overlooked, merely because it means that it's an extra expense. If we can improve our health to the point where we're not running to the doctor every five minutes, then why wouldn't we want to make that happen?

Probiotics is the topic of today's episode, but its okay if you don't know what they are. Simply put, probiotics aid in digestion, and can also help protect the overall integrity of the digestive system. Some researchers have found a direct connection between probiotics and a strong immune system, where you're less likely to get sick.

Now, that's not to say that you'll never get sick as long as you pop a probiotics pill. It's just that when you incorporate probiotics into your lifestyle, the chances of you getting majorly sick do decrease due to bacteria having less of a chance to run wild. We're really a collection of trillions and trillions of bacteria, so it makes sense that the levels "good" and "bad" bacteria matter so much. (121)

Now then, are all probiotics created equal? Not so much. If you're going to turn to probiotics to supplement your low carb lifestyle, you really need to make sure that you're also getting the highest quality probiotics around. Yogurt used to be a good probiotics staple, but the yogurts on the market do not have nearly the amount of bacterial culturing that you want. (112)

What you want to go for are lacto-fermented foods, such as kefir, sauerkraut, kimchi, lacto-fermented veggies and even lacto-fermented fruit is available. You can make all of these things at home without too much hassle. It's basically a matter of preparing the right medium and then letting time take care of the rest. Kombucha is also a very nice drink that's packed with probiotic benefit. (123)

I like the idea of going with natural sources for probiotics rather than trying to go through all of the trouble to find a suitable probiotic supplement that you can take. The more natural that you make your lifestyle, the better off you will be. Before anyone gets too tense, don't worry.

I'm still a man of science and I believe in going to the doctor. But if I can find natural ways to improve my health, then I'll look into that as well. I figure, what's the big deal, you know? If you're going to seize control of your health, then all paths have to lead to wellness, eventually.

Next episode is almost here, are you ready for it? Before we continue, I just wanted to say thank you. We're almost at the end of the series, and it means a lot to me that you're still here with me.

36 ANTIBIOTICS

Are antibiotics controversial? In the general world of low carb, not really. However, there are people who believe that antibiotics aren't doing us any favors. They do read about the rise of superbugs, and they start wondering whether or not antibiotics are really a good thing.

The reality is that antibiotics have to be viewed within the greater frame of health. There are certainly illnesses, infections, and diseases that need antibiotics. Trying to take care of strep throat (the bacterial kind) is not a good idea without antibiotics to back it up. (124)

If you're going to go with antibiotics while you're pursuing low carb, you should be aware that you're going to have to increase your intake of good bacteria. This is because when antibiotics are introduced to the body, it can wipe out the good bacteria that actually help us out, just not the bad ones. This means that all of the lovely probiotics that I mentioned in the last episode will definitely come in handy with this issue.

One thing I will address towards women is that if you're going to be on a routine of antibiotics, that you make sure to be cautious about birth control. There are studies now that indicate there is a possibility that the birth control can interact with antibiotics in ways that you may not expect. Unexpected and unintended pregnancies have occurred, which means that you will have to look at using a backup form of birth control while you're taking the antibiotics. (125)

Antibiotics are important, but they should definitely be only used for bacterial infections. Trying to take extra antibiotics that you have at home for viral infections will not do you any favors. It will simply increase the chance of drug-resistant bacteria growing out of control, in case you have another bacterial infection that you're not aware of.

Bacteria exposed to antibiotics that survive end up gaining a resistance, and that resistance has had some pretty dangerous overtones for our society as a whole. (126) I tend to use antibiotics sparingly, as should most people in my opinion. But when your doctor indicates that you're going to need antibiotics, make sure that you really know what you're taking.

The Internet is a fine resource for looking up drug information, so it's not like you can't figure out what you're taking. If you don't have immediate online access, you can always check with the pharmacist to make sure that you're not running the risk of a drug interaction. While you're feeling under the weather, you might be tempted to go off plan and give up low carb for a little while. This is definitely not something that you want to do, because it has a strong tendency of blowing up in your face.

You might think "okay, I can go off plan for a little while, and then get right back on". For some people, this is absolutely true. However, it's been my experience that once people go off plan they have to struggle for a while to get back on. There's no point in ending up this way, if you can help it.

Next episode is on its way -- how am I doing so far? Let me know -- I love hearing from my readers

37 INTERMITTENT FASTING

Now, hear me out before everyone goes nuts. I definitely think that intermittent fasting has benefits, but if you're new to low carb, you're better off doing without it. Unfortunately, so many newcomers are bombarded with differing reports and let's face it -- we all want the weight off as fast as possible.

So when someone talks about a new way to burn fat and lose weight, we're all ears. This is where people get into looking at intermittent fasting. In a nutshell, intermittent fasting is when you skip meals. You might skip breakfast, waiting until later to break your fast with what you would identify as "lunch".

Why do some people do it? Ghrelin. (127) They think about the rush of ghrelin, the hormone behind our hunger/appetite reflex in the first place. Long time intermittent fasters do indicate that they feel much more alert and focused when they're slightly hungry, compared to when they are filled with food. Is this something that is the case across the board? Absolutely not, but I think it's worth looking into under a few conditions.

First off, if you don't have a good eating pattern going

where you're getting enough calories, you need to hold off on intermittent fasting. This is even more the case if you're suffering from adrenal fatigue. This isn't the time to get involved with IF, because you are going to be inviting new stresses into the body.

Next, if you've struggled with disordered eating in the past, IF can be a ticket to a lot of headaches for you. This is something that would be better to avoid more than anything else.

You definitely want to make sure that your mindset is focused on getting the best out of IF, not the worst out of it. It's all about fretting up the right feeding window (128). If you're going to try IF'ing for the first time, make sure that you go with a short fasting window to start with.

Starting with a long 18 hour window isn't a good idea at all -- it's just going to make you frustrated if you can't last that long. Starting with a 12 hour fast and moving up gradually to a 14 and then a 16 hour one is the better approach.

Keep in mind that this is just for those that really want to optimize their fat loss journey. There's nothing in the world that says that you have to go with the intermittent fasting thing at all. You can always switch gears, go with something different, and make sure that your needs are covered by low carb eating and moderate exercise.

Just because you go into this fasting protocol doesn't mean that you have to necessarily give up everything else. Indeed, sleep will still be important, stress management will be highly important, and you will still want to remain strictly on plan (129).

If you can do that, then you'll find some benefits with intermittent fasting. I tend to also caution it with women, because the risk for hormonal imbalance and possible adrenal fatigue can rise up. Since everyone is different, you'll have to see for yourself.

38 CAFFEINE

Uh oh, I might be trampling on someone's sacred ground here, because this episode is all about caffeine. You see, I don't think caffeine should be a free for all type of thing if you're on a low carb diet. You need to encourage yourself to limit caffeine intake, for a wide variety of reasons.

As you might already know, caffeine is a stimulant, and too much stimulant can definitely be a bad thing. If you're getting to the point where you're constantly powered by caffeine, you might have bigger problems than you think. (130)

According to the Mayo Clinic, two to four cups of coffee a day isn't that bad. However, a lot of people ignore the caffeine in chocolate, tea, coffee, and energy drinks. If you're constantly using caffeine to prop you up, you have an addiction to caffeine that could be impacting your health.

It's nothing to get immediately alarmed about -- many people rely on caffeine and other stimulants to get from one day to the next. But the problem with doing that is that you never really give your body the chance it needs to rest and recover. You definitely want to make sure that you're avoiding extra stress on the body during your low carb lifestyle, as I've said in a few episodes. (1, continued)

Another reason to avoid caffeine is that if you have unstable blood sugar, there's a possibility that it can trigger more blood sugar instability problems. Even if you're in ketosis, you still have to think about this issue [Note: I touched on ketosis in Episode #30] carefully. Speaking of ketosis, if you start giving into cravings triggered by an erratic blood sugar spike, your chances of staying in ketosis are very slim unless you pick foods that are already on plan.

Generally speaking, when people feel their blood sugar beginning to spiral out of control, they really don't think about whether something is low carb or not. They just reach for it, and then regret it later. Once you start regretting your choices, you tend to continue to make bad choices because you feel that the day is ruined. Over time, this leads to weight gain. Not always, of course, but in most people, the extra pounds tend to creep back on.

There are some benefits of caffeine in workouts (131) that are good to know about. For one, you're giving yourself a burst of energy, which can be helpful when you're trying to move your routine to a much tougher one. The more that you can do on your own, the better off you will feel -- but sometimes everyone needs a little pick me up, you know?

My focus here is to give you good information that you can use for the long haul. If there's anything that I haven't covered, you can always send me a note. Caffeine is one of those things that you just can't talk to people about without seeing how passionate they really are. Most people would honestly give up their cell phones before they would give up coffee.

If you're going to be a low carb rockstar, make sure that you avoid sugar in your cup of coffee. Get heavy whipping cream, butter, anything but the dreaded white stuff.

Speaking of the white stuff, let's get ready for the next episode: all about sweeteners!

39 SWEETENERS

Are all sweeteners the same? Definitely not. If you're low carbing, then you've probably been warned all about the dangers of sugar. Sugar in this case is that granulated white stuff that's on kitchen counters, restaurants and even in bars. If you want to get healthy, you have to avoid sugar.

That can be hard, considering that it's in just about everything you can think of. Even some low carb items use sweetness to boost their appeal, and that's not a good thing. Sugar affects the liver and how it filters toxins, which is just one more reason to avoid sugar. (132)

But if you're looking at your low carb lifestyle and craving a little sweetness, you don't have to give up -- you can always move on to actual low carb. One of the newest ones would have to be monkfruit. This is actually a low carb sweetener, and you don't have to use much in order to really capture a sweet flavor.

Monkfruit is also known as Luo Han Guo. Be careful if you decide to go with Nectresse, which is a sweetener marketed as low-carb. While it's technically low carb, you should be aware that it uses molasses as well as sugar in the packets, though in very small amounts.

There's also stevia, which has been used for thousands of years. There are stevia product son the market, from liquid drops all the way up to powdered varieties. Some people even grow stevia right in little herb pots on their kitchen windowsill.

The freshest stevia leads to good sweetness, but in terms of convenience, you can really beat having little packets that you can take with you. Most restaurants will have some type of sweetener, but it might not be low carb.

The most popular type of stevia on the market right now is actually a blend called Truvia, which cuts down on stevia's infamous bitter aftertaste. It's up to you whether you want to use Truvia or Pruvia. Some people are staunchly against these products, while others feel that they're okay, but they would prefer going with more natural sources of sweetness. (133)

They could have Splenda, known as sucralose in generic terms. Splenda tastes very similar to sugar and can be used in baking very easily. There is a bit of a cooling effect in the mouth from time to time, but most low carb fans report that Splenda is really their go-to sweetener of choice.

Another sweetener that is really popular is xylitol -- it's actually a sugar alcohol, which means that it's a substance that has a lesser impact on insulin than full out sugar. You want to be careful of getting too excited by sugar alcohols, as they can cause digestive upset if you eat too many of them. (134)

Some people choose to go without sweetener. I tend to do without sweetener for most things, but I've lasso been low carb for a while. If you're new to low carbing then chances are good you'll want some sweetness in your diet.

Over time though, don't be surprised that your taste buds change to the point where you really don't crave that type of sweetness anymore. Everyone will have to make their own decisions -- but I think there's still room at the low carb table for everyone. Why not look into these sweeteners on your own? You might try to get some sample bottles of each one, so you can figure out what your personal tastes are. Our final episode is right around the corner.

40 IGNORING THE THYROID

Well, we're at the end of the series -- did you get anything out of the episodes? I really hope so, because this health business is my passion. I want each and every one of you to reach for better health, start feeling good and really digging deeply into your new life. Low carb isn't just something to do for a little while. I need you to make it your lifestyle, and I've tried to include as much information as I could for you to make that choice.

One area that low carbers tend to ignore at first would be the thyroid, but this isn't a good idea at all. The truth is that the thyroid has a lot of function within the body. You literally cannot go without the thyroid -- and you will have to be placed on special medication if you lost complete thyroid function.

People who struggle with weight due to an underperforming thyroid most likely suffer from hypothyroidism, if not full blown Hashimoto's Thyroiditis. Hypothyroidism is when the thyroid underperforms, but you might not know what the symptoms really are. Generally speaking, you can deal with a lot less stamina and energy than what others in your age range would experience.

If you're in your early 20s but you feel like you're 50, you might have some problems with your thyroid. If you can't really lift your arms after activity, you could have problems with your thyroid. And if you have depression that just doesn't seem to go away, you might have problems with your thyroid. (135)

Other thyroid issues revolve around temperature -- being either too hot (hyperthyroidism) or too cold (hypothyroidism). The thyroid plays a role in other hormones as well, so generally speaking if your thyroid is having problems, other hormone levels will be off as well.

Now that we know what we're up against, what's the best solution? A low carb diet. No, really, it's true. Those that suffer from hypothyroidism find that a low carb diet helps them feel satisfied without weighing them down, and it can help ease the symptoms of an underperforming thyroid.

However, supplementation may still be in order. Many with these issues still turn to desiccated thyroid from quality sources, or they add in iodine through kelp flakes, seaweed, and other good low carb sources of iodine. Both can help when it comes to a thyroid that isn't producing enough hormone to keep you moving forward. (136)

If you suspect that you're having problems with your thyroid, only a doctor can officially diagnose your symptoms. I strongly suggest making an appointment. If your levels are not up to par and you're really in the severe zone, you could have an autoimmune disorder known as Hashimoto's Thyroiditis.

It's nothing to joke about or take lightly, as it attacks the whole body -- not just the thyroid. There are people that have developed serious health conditions by ignoring the thyroid issues that they already had. Everything in your body is linked, after all. (137)

The more that you can focus on your health, the better.

This is the last episode for the time being, so I really hope you enjoyed them all. As always, if something doesn't make sense to you, just feel free to drop me a line and we'll discuss it together. After all, that's what I'm here for. Take care!

REFERENCES

1. http://blogs.webmd.com/pamela-peeke-md/2010/04/dieting-is-stressful-ditch-the-diet-mentality.html

2. http://www.webmd.com/diet/news/20090708/lifes-stress-may-lead-to-weight-gain

3. http://www.ncbi.nlm.nih.gov/pubmed/2166857

4. http://donmatesz.blogspot.com/2011/05/nutrient-density-of-dietary-fats-and.html

5. http://articles.mercola.com/sites/articles/archive/2010/04/20/sugar-dangers.aspx

6. http://www.ncbi.nlm.nih.gov/pubmed/8622814

7. http://www.livingpaleo.com/foods-to-avoid-on-the-paleo-diet/

8. http://healthysleep.med.harvard.edu/healthy/matters/benefits-of-sleep/why-do-we-sleep

9. http://www.ncbi.nlm.nih.gov/pubmed/6741850

10. http://www.webmd.com/diet/healthtool-metabolism-calculator

11. http://www.webmd.com/diet/calories-chart

12 http://lowcarbdiets.about.com/od/lowcarb101/a/firstweek.htm

13http://authoritynutrition.com/7-reasons-not-to-have-cheat-meals-or-days/

14. http://www.webmd.com/diet/tc/obesity-health-risks-of-obesity

15. http://www.naturalmedicinejournal.com/article_content.asp?article=93

16. http://www.sleepfoundation.org/article/how-sleep-works/how-much-sleep-do-we-really-need

17. http://www.mayoclinic.com/health/sleep/HQ01387

18. http://www.sleepforall.com/sleep-cycle.htm

19. http://healthland.time.com/2013/02/08/sleeping-it-off-how-alcohol-affects-sleep-quality/

20. http://www.sciencelearn.org.nz/Contexts/Uniquely-Me/Science-Ideas-and-Concepts/Role-of-proteins-in-the-body

21. http://www.huffingtonpost.com/dr-mercola/soy-health_b_1822466.html

22. http://www.webmd.com/food-recipes/protein

23. http://www.medicinenet.com/script/main/art.asp?articlekey=50900

24. http://lowcarbdiets.about.com/od/whattoeat/a/alcbev.htm

25. http://www2.potsdam.edu/hansondj/HealthIssues/1110385823.html

26. http://www.psychologytoday.com/blog/addiction-in-society/201011/science-is-what-society-says-it-is-alcohols-poison

27. https://www.getfit.tn.gov/kids/calories.aspx

28 http://www.calorieking.com/foods/

29. http://www.ncbi.nlm.nih.gov/pubmed/16001844

30 http://perfecthealthdiet.com/2010/11/dangers-of-zero-carb-diets-i-can-there-be-a-carbohydrate-deficiency/

31 Aiello LC, Wheeler P. The expensive tissue hypothesis: the brain and the digestive system in human and primate evolution. Current Anthropology 1995(Apr); 36(2):199-211.

32 http://www.ncbi.nlm.nih.gov/pubmed/17621514?dopt=AbstractPlus

33 http://www.ncbi.nlm.nih.gov/pubmed/5919366?dopt=AbstractPlus

34. http://www.ncbi.nlm.nih.gov/pmc/articles/PMC2784228/

35. http://www.mayoclinic.com/health/exercise/HQ01676

36. http://www.huffingtonpost.com/2013/03/27/mental-health-benefits-exercise_n_2956099.html

37.http://www.naturalnews.com/007842_physical_exercise_preventing_diabetes.
html

38. http://www.huffingtonpost.com/dr-mark-hyman/food-
allergy_b_1301271.html

39. http://www.huffingtonpost.com/chris-kresser/gluten-
intolerance_b_2964812.html

40. http://www.webmd.com/allergies/guide/allergies-elimination-diet

41. http://news.sciencemag.org/sciencenow/2012/05/silent-killer-may-be-
disease-of-.html

42. Jacobs, Jürgen. "Quantitative measurement of food selection." Oecologia 14.4
(1974): 413-417.

43. http://www.kpchr.org/research/public/News.aspx?NewsID=3

44. http://www.fitday.com

45. http://www.myfitnesspal.com

46. http://www.huffingtonpost.com/william-anderson-ma-lmhc/weight-loss-
advice_b_3116384.html

47. http://www.healthdiscovery.net/articles/scale_lies.htm

48. http://www.livestrong.com/article/418602-how-to-change-your-mindset-to-
lose-weight/

49. http://www.shapeup.org/bfl/bioelec.html

50.
http://www.cnn.com/2011/HEALTH/expert.q.a/09/30/body.fat.testing.jampoli
s/index.html

51. http://www.mayoclinic.com/health/weight-loss-plateau/MY01152

52. http://www-rohan.sdsu.edu/~ens304l/skinfold.htm

53. http://www.mayoclinic.com/health/stress/sr00001

54. http://www.health.harvard.edu/newsweek/Understanding_Cholesterol.htm

55 http://www.hsph.harvard.edu/nutritionsource/fats-full-story/

56 http://wellnessmama.com/5356/cravings-fix-your-leptin/

57. http://lewrockwell.com/mercola/mercola177.html

58. http://www.doctoroz.com/videos/surprising-health-benefits-coconut-oil

59. http://articles.mercola.com/sites/articles/archive/2013/01/17/avocado-benefits.aspx

60. http://paleodietlifestyle.com/the-many-virtues-of-butter/

61. http://www.ncbi.nlm.nih.gov/pubmed/21310306

62. http://www.naturalnews.com/036181_blacks_vitamin_D_deficiency_cancer.html

63. http://www.proteinpower.com/drmike/saturated-fat/tips-tricks-for-starting-or-restarting-low-carb-pt-ii/

64. http://soils.usda.gov/use/worldsoils/papers/land-degradation-overview.html

65. http://www.amarillomed.com/howto

66. http://anaemic.org/anemia-in-men.php

67. http://www.diabetes.org/living-with-diabetes/complications/

68. http://men.webmd.com/features/low-testosterone-explained-how-do-you-know-when-levels-are-too-low

69. http://www.diabetes.org/food-and-fitness/fitness/weight-loss/setting-realistic-weight-loss.html

70. http://diets.ultimatefatburner.com/stop-cheating-carb-diet/

71 http://pureathletefitness.com/pics

72. http://www.health.am/ab/more/packaged-foods-and-obesity/

73. http://www.mayoclinic.com/health/monosodium-glutamate/AN01251

74. http://www.nutrition.gov/shopping-cooking-meal-planning/food-shopping-and-meal-planning/farmers-markets

75. http://www.ncbi.nlm.nih.gov/pubmed/22825366

76. http://www.grainstorm.com/pages/modern-wheat

77. http://www.centerimt.com/gluten-elimination-diet.php

78 http://www.huffingtonpost.com/dr-mark-hyman/gluten-what-you-dont-know_b_379089.html

79. http://www.news-medical.net/health/Testosterone-Physiological-Effects.aspx

80. http://www.nlm.nih.gov/medlineplus/tutorials/lowtestosterone/ur189103.pdf

81. http://jap.physiology.org/content/82/1/49.full

82. http://www.news-medical.net/health/Estrogen-What-is-Estrogen.aspx

83. http://www.womentowomen.com/menopause/estrogendominance.aspx

84. http://www.nih.gov/news/health/aug2010/nichd-10.htm

85. http://www.lookcut.com/articles/cortisol-weight-loss-myths.html

86. http://www.sciencedaily.com/releases/2006/09/060918142456.htm

87. http://eurheartj.oxfordjournals.org/cgi/content/full/29/15/1903

88. http://www.livestrong.com/article/412216-will-bananas-raise-blood-sugar/

89. http://healthyfitmom.com/potassium-rich-low-carb-foods/

90. http://www.emedicinehealth.com/low_potassium/article_em.htm

91. http://www.fitday.com/fitness-articles/nutrition/vitamins-minerals/potassium-why-its-essential-for-your-body.html

92. http://www.healthyandorganic.com/magnesium.html

93. Rubin H. Central role for magnesium in coordinate control of metabolism and growth in animal cells. Proceedings of the National Academy of Sciences of the USA. 1975 Sep;72(9):3551-5.

94. http://www.medscape.com/viewarticle/423568

95. http://journals.lww.com/acsm-msse/Fulltext/2009/03000/Progression_Models_in_Resistance_Training_for.26.aspx

96. http://www.mayoclinic.com/health/strength-training/HQ01710

97. http://breakingmuscle.com/strength-conditioning/proof-pull-10-tools-getting-better-pull-ups

98. TABATA, I. et al. (1996) Effects of moderate-intensity endurance and high-intensity intermittent training on anaerobic capacity and VO2max. Med Sci Sports Exerc., 28 (10), p. 1327-1330.

99. Gorostiaga, E.M., et al. Uniqueness of interval and continuous training at the same maintained exercise intensity. European Journal of Applied Physiology 63(2):101-107, 1991.

100. King, J.W. A comparison of the effects of interval training vs. continuous training on weight loss and body composition in obese premenopausal women (thesis). East Tennessee State University, 2001.

101. Meuret, J.R., et al. A comparison of the effects of continuous aerobic, intermittent aerobic, and resistance exercise on resting metabolic rate at 12 and 21 hours post-exercise. Medicine & Science in Sports & Exercise 39(5 suppl):S247, 2007.

102. http://www.choosemyplate.gov/food-groups/fruits-why.html

103. http://www.webmd.com/food-recipes/features/how-antioxidants-work1

104. http://lowcarbdiets.about.com/od/whattoeat/a/whatfruit.htm

105. http://www.medicalnewstoday.com/articles/180858.php

106. Leung, L.H. "Pantothetic acid as a weight reducing agent: fasting without hunger, weakness and ketosis". Medical Hypothesis. 44(5):403-5 May, 1995.

107. Vazquez, Jorje, and S. Adibi. "Protein sparing during treatment of obesity:

110

ketogenic versus nonketogenic very low calorie diet". Metabolism. 41(4): 406-414, April 1994.

108 http://www.organicconsumers.org/nutricon/qa.cfm

109 http://abcnews.go.com/blogs/health/2012/06/01/high-protein-low-carb-diet-safe-for-kidneys/

110 http://www.mayoclinic.com/health/diabetic-ketoacidosis/DS00674/DSECTION=symptoms

111 http://slowburnfitness.com/ketosis-vs-ketoacidosis/

112 http://www.ncbi.nlm.nih.gov/pmc/articles/PMC2129159/

113 http://www.doctoroz.com/videos/five-ways-fight-inflammation

114 Childers N.F. A relationship of arthritis to the Solanaceae (nightshades). J Intern Acad Prev Med 1979; 7:31-37

115 http://www.mayoclinic.com/health/adrenal-fatigue/AN01583

116 http://robbwolf.com/2012/04/09/real-deal-adrenal-fatigue/

117 http://www.tvernonlac.com/adrenal-fatigue-diet.html

118 http://chriskresser.com/how-too-much-omega-6-and-not-enough-omega-3-is-making-us-sick

119 http://www.kumc.edu/school-of-medicine/integrative-medicine/health-topics/healthy-cooking-oils.html

120 http://www.westonaprice.org/cod-liver-oil/cod-liver-oil-setting-the-record-straight

121 http://www.webmd.com/digestive-disorders/tc/probiotics-topic-overview

122 http://www.aafp.org/afp/2008/1101/p1073.html

123 http://www.nourishedlivingnetwork.com/recipe-photo-gallery/living-and-lacto-fermented-foods/

124 http://www.mayoclinic.com/health/antibiotics/FL00075

125
http://student.ahc.umn.edu/dental/coursearchives/3yr_Summer/DENT5701/A
ntibiotics%20and%20Oral%20Contraception.pdf

126 http://www.nlm.nih.gov/medlineplus/antibiotics.html

127 http://www.romanfitnesssystems.com/blog/intermittent-fasting-101/

128 http://www.gnolls.org/79/i-am-a-ghrelin-addict/

129 http://syattfitness.com/nutrition/intermittent-fasting-it-might-not-be-right-
for-you-and-thats-o-k/

130 http://www.mayoclinic.com/health/caffeine/NU00600

131 http://livinlavidalocarb.blogspot.com/2007/08/does-caffeine-impact-ketosis-
on-low.html

132 http://www.nytimes.com/2011/04/17/magazine/mag-17Sugar-
t.html?pagewanted=all

133 http://www.lowcarb.ca/tips/tips006.html

134 http://www.kitchenstewardship.com/2012/02/17/xylitol-erythritol-
sorbitolwhats-that-ol-about/

135 http://www.mayoclinic.com/health/hypothyroidism/DS00353

136 http://jcem.endojournals.org/content/85/9/3191.short

137 http://thyroid.about.com/od/gettestedanddiagnosed/a/testdiagnose.htm

ABOUT THE AUTHOR

Mirsad writes all of his books in a unique style, constantly drawing connections between his past failures and the student's goals, so that you can avoid experiencing the same frustrations that he did. He doesn't promise you the world, but what he does promise you is that if you follow his tips and advice, you will reach your goals, guaranteed!

Made in the USA
Lexington, KY
12 May 2014